Dental Radiography
Laboratory Manual

Dental Radiography
Laboratory Manual

SANDRA SLACK OLSON, RDH, MEd, CAGS

Professor, Dental Hygiene Department
Quinsigamond Community College
Worcester, Massachusetts

W. B. SAUNDERS COMPANY

A Division of Harcourt Brace & Company
PHILADELPHIA   LONDON   TORONTO   MONTREAL   SYDNEY   TOKYO

W. B. SAUNDERS COMPANY
A Division of Harcourt Brace & Company

The Curtis Center
Independence Square West
Philadelphia, PA   19106

Library of Congress Cataloging-in-Publication Data

Olson, Sandra Slack,
    Dental radiography laboratory manual/Sandra Slack Olson.
      p. cm.
    ISBN 0-7216-6455-5
    1. Teeth—Radiography—Laboratory manuals. I. Title.
    [DNLM: 1. Radiography, Dental—laboratory manuals. WU 25 052d
1994]
    RK309.044 1995
    617.6'07572—dc20
    DNLM/DLC

                94-8369

DENTAL RADIOGRAPHY LABORATORY MANUAL   ISBN   0-7216-6455-5

Printed in the United States of America.

Last digit is the print number: 9   8   7   6   5   4   3   2

This book is dedicated

in loving memory of my mother,

Daisy Scofield Slack

and

to my daughter,

Annalisa Olson

Preface

Dental Radiography Laboratory Manual has been designed to supplement available radiography texts. The purpose of this manual is to review the material in a simple manner that will be easily understood by the student. Each chapter begins with learning objectives that describe what the student should know after completing the chapter. Learning activities and review questions for the lab, home, and classroom conclude each chapter and assist the student in achieving the chapter's objectives.

Since it is in the laboratory that dental hygiene and dental assisting students learn the radiographic technique, processing, infection control, and patient management skills required in their profession, it is also the purpose of this manual to provide laboratory exercises and activities that assist the student in mastering the technical skills required to produce radiographs of optimum quality with minimum discomfort and radiation exposure to the patient.

This manual is designed to be "user-friendly" for both students and educators. The sequencing of the chapters may be altered to adapt to the needs and format of individual radiography courses. Laboratory exercises appropriate to your course should be selected and adapted as needed. Some of the exercises can form the basis for a demonstration or collaborative group learning activity for the students. Be creative in your use of the material.

I would like to express my thanks to Professor Paul Connell for his assistance with the production of photographs for this manual and for his humor and moral support. Thanks as well go to Daniel La Marche for the production of the photographs of radiographs in the manual. I would also like to thank my father, Bradley Slack, and my friends and neighbors, Joanne and Hank Fitzgerald, for their support and help during its preparation. Finally, I would like to thank my students for helping me to be a better teacher.

SANDRA SLACK OLSON

Contents

Radiation Hazards and Protection

LEARNING OBJECTIVES

After completing this chapter the student will be able to

1. Describe basic atomic structure, including
   Nucleus
   Neutron, proton, and electron
   Orbital shells
   Binding energy
2. Describe ionization.
3. Describe particulate and electromagnetic radiation.
4. Identify radiations in the electromagnetic spectrum.
5. List the characteristics of electromagnetic radiations.
6. Describe the significance of the wavelength of electromagnetic radiations.
7. Describe the results of the interaction of x rays with matter.
8. Describe the direct and indirect effects of ionizing radiation.
9. List three types of biologic damage which may result from exposure to ionizing radiation.
10. List and describe factors which influence the biologic effect of radiation.
11. List factors which influence radiosensitivity and identify radiosensitive cells and organs.
12. Describe the ALARA concept.
13. Describe the protection provided to the patient by the Consumer Health and Safety Act of 1981.
14. Use the Department of Health and Human Services' guidelines for prescribing radiographs in determining a patient's need for radiographs.
15. Describe equipment factors which influence radiation exposure.
16. Describe the influence of film speed on radiation exposure.

17. Describe the influence of exposure and processing techniques on radiation exposure.

18. Describe effective procedures for radiation protection for an operator.

19. Describe methods of monitoring radiation exposure to operators.

20. Define the following terms:

Atom	Maximum permissible dose (MPD)
Attenuation	
Binding energy	Molecule
Collimation	Neutron
Coulomb per kilogram (C/kg)	Nucleus
	Primary radiation
Dose	Proton
Dose rate	Radiation
Drift	Radiation absorbed dose (rad)
Electron	
Element	Radiosensitivity
Exposure	Roentgen (R)
Filtration	Roentgen equivalent man (rem)
Gray (Gy)	
Head leakage	Scatter radiation
Ionization	Secondary radiation
Ion pair	Seivert (Sv)
Joule	Total dose

I. BASIC ATOMIC STRUCTURE

Before describing methods of protecting the patient and operator from exposure to ionizing radiation, it is necessary to review some basic concepts of atomic structure and the interaction of x rays with matter.

A. Elements

An **element** is a simple substance made up of atoms having the same atomic number and the same chemical properties.

B. Atoms

An **atom** is the smallest particle of an element that retains the properties of the element (Fig. 1-1).

The **nucleus** of the atom is a heavy inner core containing subatomic particles called **neutrons** and **protons.** Protons are positively charged, and there is a specific number of them for each element. This number determines the atomic number of the element. Neutrons have no charge and are neutral.

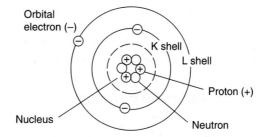

Figure 1-1. A diagram of a lithium atom. The nucleus contains neutrons and protons. Since there are three protons, lithium has an atomic number of 3. The number of electrons orbiting around the nucleus in shells equals the number of protons.

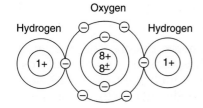

Figure 1-2. A water molecule. A molecule is made up of more than one atom. It is the smallest particle of a substance that retains the chemical properties of that substance.

Electrons are negatively charged subatomic particles that travel around the nucleus in orbits called *shells.* The shells vary in distance from the nucleus and are labeled *k, l, m, n, o, p,* and *q* from the shell closest to the nucleus to the most distant.

The **binding energy** that holds the electrons in place in their orbits is a balance of the centrifugal force of the orbiting electrons, which repels them from the nucleus, and the positive charge of the protons, which attracts them. The binding energy is strongest with electrons closest to the nucleus in the *k* shell. In an electrically neutral or stable atom, the number of electrons equals the number of protons.

C. Molecules

A **molecule** is made up of more than one atom (Fig. 1-2). It is the smallest particle of a substance that still retains the physical and chemical properties of the substance.

D. Ionization

Ionization occurs when an electron is removed from an electrically neutral atom (Fig. 1-3). This creates a *positive ion,* an atom that is positively charged, and a *free electron,* which is negatively charged. Together they are called an **ion pair.**

Figure 1-3. Ionization occurs when an electron is removed from an electrically neutral atom. This creates a positive ion, an atom that is positively charged, and a free electron, which is negatively charged. Together they are called an *ion pair.*

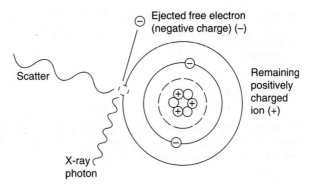

For ionization to occur, sufficient energy must be introduced to overcome the binding energy of the electron. Inner-shell electrons can only be displaced by x rays, gamma rays, or high-energy particles. Outer-shell electrons are more easily displaced.

II. TYPES OF RADIATION

Radiation is the transmission of energy through space and matter. It is emitted from atoms as they go through internal change. There are two types of radiation.

A. Particulate Radiation

Particulate radiation is the transmission of kinetic energy (the energy of motion) by subatomic particles emitted at high speeds by unstable atoms. Examples of particulate radiation are beta rays, which are high-speed electrons emitted from radioactive nuclei, and cathode rays, which are high-speed electrons created in a machine (the high-speed electrons within the x-ray tube).

B. Electromagnetic Radiation

Electromagnetic radiation is the movement of energy through space as a combination of electrical and magnetic energy. It is created when the speed of an electrically charged particle is changed. Gamma rays are naturally occurring electromagnetic radiations similar to x rays which originate in the nucleus of radioactive atoms. X rays are man-made radiations originating in machines. Other forms of electromagnetic radiation include light, radio, and television waves, electricity, and ultraviolet rays (Fig. 1-4).

All electromagnetic radiations travel at the speed of light (186,000 mi/s) in a wave-like motion, have electrical and magnetic fields, and have measurable and different energies.

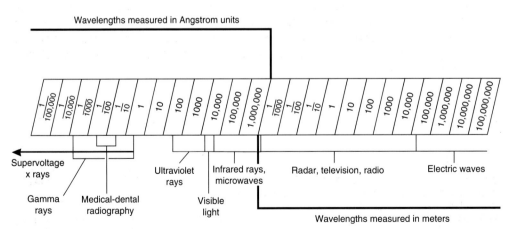

Figure 1-4. The electromagnetic spectrum. Lower-energy radiations such as electricity and television waves have longer wavelengths. High-energy radiations such as x rays and ultraviolet rays have shorter wavelengths.

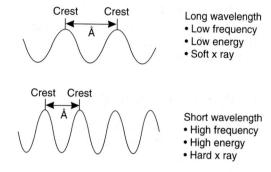

Figure 1-5. Wavelength is measured by determining the distance between the wave crests. Radiations with shorter wavelengths have more energy than those with longer wavelengths. Long-wavelength radiations are measured in centimeters, while short-wavelength radiations such as x rays are measured in angstrom units.

The energy of electromagnetic radiation is determined by its *wavelength*. Wavelength is measured by determining the distance between the wave crests. Radiations with shorter wavelengths have more energy than those with longer wavelengths (Fig. 1-5). Long-wavelength radiations are measured in centimeters, while short-wavelength radiations such as x rays are measured in angstrom units.

III. X RADIATION

Dental x rays are produced in a tube by converting the kinetic energy of high-speed electrons to heat and x-ray energy (see Chap. 3). The individual units of x-ray energy emitted from the tube are called *photons.* Photons vary in wavelength and, therefore, have varying amounts of energy.

Primary radiation is the radiation that emerges from the x-ray machine before it interacts with matter. **Secondary** or **scatter radiation** is that which results from the interaction of x rays with matter (Fig. 1-6).

A. The Interaction of X Rays with Matter

The following are the result of the interaction of x rays with matter:

❐ **Attenuation** is a reduction in the number of x-ray photons in the x-ray beam. This occurs when x-ray photons give up all their energy and are absorbed by matter. The degree of attenuation or absorption depends on the energy of the photons and the thickness and density of the absorbing material.

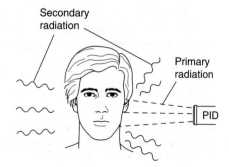

Figure 1-6. Primary radiation is the radiation that emerges from the x-ray machine before it interacts with matter. Secondary or scatter radiation is that which results from the interaction of x rays with matter.

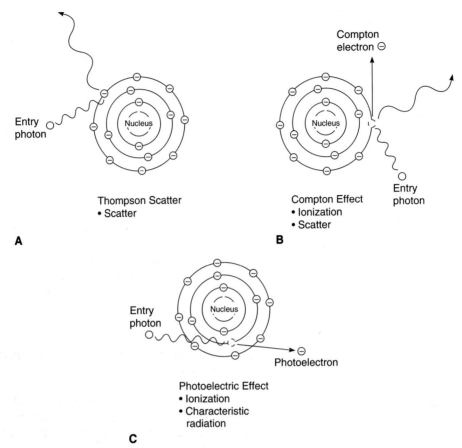

Figure 1-7. The interaction of x rays with matter. **(A)** Thompson scatter. An x-ray photon passes near an outer-shell electron, causing it to vibrate and give off secondary radiation. **(B)** The Compton effect. An electron is removed from an outer shell, and the photon is deflected from its path. This results in ionization and scattered radiation. **(C)** The photoelectric effect. An inner-shell electron is ejected from its shell, causing ionization. Outer-shell electrons move into inner shells to replace the vacancy. This movement creates secondary radiation with a wavelength characteristic of the binding energy of the atom.

☐ **Secondary** or **scatter radiation** is produced when an x-ray photon interacts with an atom and creates new radiation or is deflected from its path. Because some of the original energy of the photon is given up in the interaction, secondary or scatter radiation has less energy than primary radiation (Fig. 1-7).

☐ **Ionization** occurs when an x-ray photon strikes an orbiting electron in an atom and ejects it from its shell (Fig. 1-7B,C). The molecules of living organisms are composed of atoms that can be ionized by radiation. Ionization may alter the molecule, causing damage to the organism.

IV. RADIATION MEASUREMENT

To measure a quantity of something, a unit of measurement must be used. To measure distance, Americans have traditionally used inches, feet, yards, and miles as the units of measurement. To standardize distance measurement internationally, the metric system is used. The metric units of measurement for distance are the millimeter, centimeter, meter, and kilometer. When discussing radiation hazards and protection, exposure, dose, and dose equivalent are measured. They have traditionally been measured using the older units of measurement: roentgen, rad, and rem. The newer units of measurement recommended to standardize radiation measurement internationally are Systems International, or SI, units.

A. Exposure

Exposure is a measurement of the quantity of radiation to which an object or organism is *subjected.* Some of this radiation will be absorbed, and some will pass through the organism. Exposure is measured by identifying the amount of ionization produced in air by *x* or *gamma radiation.* An *ionization chamber* is used for this purpose (Fig. 1-8). The units of measurement for exposure are as follows:

❐ **Roentgen (R)** is the traditional unit of measurement. It is the amount of radiation that will produce 2.08 × 10 ion pairs in a cubic centimeter of air at a standard pressure and temperature.

❐ **Coulomb per kilogram (C/kg)** is the Systeme International (SI) unit. A coulomb is a unit of measurement of electrical charge. The coulomb per kilogram measures electrical charges (ion pairs) in a kilogram of air. 1 C/kg = 3.88×10^3 R or 1 C/kg = 3888 R.

B. Absorbed Dose

The amount of *any type* of radiation energy *absorbed* by matter is the absorbed **dose.** The **joule (J)** is a unit of energy measurement. Absorbed dose measures the amount energy (joules) deposited in an object. The units of measurement of dose are as follows:

❐ **Radiation absorbed dose (rad)** is the traditional unit of measurement of dose. A rad is the absorption of 0.01 J/kg of matter.

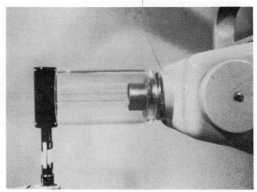

Figure 1-8. An ionization chamber measures exposure by identifying the amount of ionization produced in air by *x* or *gamma radiation.* (From Frommer HH: *Radiology for Dental Auxiliaries,* 5th ed. St. Louis, Mosby–Year Book, 1992, p. 48.)

Table 1-1. Sample Rem Calculations

Radiation	Absorbed Dose	×	QF	=	Dose Equivalent
X rays	5 rad	×	1	=	5 rem
Gamma rays	5 rad	×	1	=	5 rem
Protons	5 rad	×	10	=	50 rem
Alpha particles	5 rad	×	20	=	100 rem

Table 1-2. Sample Sv Calculations (SI)

Radiation	Absorbed Dose	×	QF	=	Dose Equivalent
X rays	5 Gy	×	1	=	5 Sv
Gamma rays	5 Gy	×	1	=	5 Sv
Protons	5 Gy	×	10	=	50 Sv
Alpha particles	5 Gy	×	20	=	100 Sv

❐ **The Gray (Gy)** is the SI unit that measures dose. One Gray equals the absorption of 1 J/kg of matter. Also, 1 Gy = 100 rad.

C. Dose Equivalent

The harmful effects of doses of *various types of ionizing radiations* may be compared using *dose equivalent.* The same absorbed dose of x rays and gamma rays produces the same effect in body tissues. However, a dose of other ionizing radiation such as neutrons, protons, or alpha particles produces a greater biologic effect than the same dose of x or gamma radiation. Dose equivalent is the product of the absorbed dose times a biologic effect qualifying factor. The units of measurement of dose equivalent are as follows:

❐ **Roentgen equivalent man (rem)** is the traditional unit of measurement of dose equivalent. One rem equals 1 rad times the qualifying factor (QF) for the type of ionizing radiation absorbed (Table 1-1).

❐ The **sievert (Sv)** is the SI unit that measures dose equivalent. One sievert equals 1 Gy times the qualifying factor (QF) for the type of ionizing radiation absorbed (Table 1-2).

When measuring dental radiation:

$$R = rad = rem \text{ and a } C/kg = Gy = Sv.$$

V. BIOLOGIC EFFECTS OF RADIATION

Biologic damage from radiation occurs on three levels: molecular, cellular, and organic. When atoms composing the molecules of living tissues are ionized, they will no longer bond properly into molecules. Damaged molecules can alter the chemical balance of the cell and impair cellular functioning.

A. Direct Effects

Ionizing radiation may interact directly with macromolecules (DNA, RNA, proteins, enzymes) causing the breakage of chemical bonds and the creation of abnormal structures. When this occurs, the damage is a *direct effect* of the radiation. DNA is the most sensitive molecule to radiation damage. While most of the damage may be repaired, unrepaired damage may accumulate proportionally with each radiation exposure. Damaged DNA may transmit the wrong genetic message.

B. Indirect Effects

When water is ionized, chemicals may be created that cause biologic damage. Biologic damage caused by these chemicals is an *indirect effect* of ionizing radiation. Most of the effects of ionizing radiation in the body are indirect.

C. Types of Biologic Damage

There are three types of biologic damage that may result from exposure to ionizing radiation:

❐ *Cell death* may occur. While this is the desired result in radiation therapy, it can have disastrous results on a developing embryo. The major embryonic effect of exposure to ionizing radiation is mental retardation.

❐ *Mutations* may occur in germ cells which will have genetic consequences in later generations. This does not result in new mutations but rather in an increase in the number of mutations that already occur spontaneously.

❐ *Carcinogenesis* or *leukemogenesis* may occur. With any exposure to ionizing radiation, a cancer cell may be produced. This may result in the development of leukemia or other cancers. Leukemia has the shortest latency (the period between exposure and clinical evidence of the disease). Solid tumors have a latency of 20 to 40 years.

D. Influencing Factors

The following factors influence the biologic effects of ionizing radiation:

❐ **Total dose** is the total amount of ionizing radiation absorbed by a patient. Larger doses of radiation cause more damage.

❐ **Dose rate** is the period of time during which the total dose occurs. A specific dose of radiation spread out over a long period of time will cause less damage than the same dose given in a short period of time because it allows time for the repair of radiation damage.

❐ *Localized versus whole-body dose* is a factor. A *localized dose* of radiation occurs only in a specific area, while a *whole-body dose* occurs in the entire body. A dose of radiation to the whole body is more damaging than the same dose confined to a specific area.

Table 1-3. Tissue Sensitivity

High Sensitivity	Moderate Sensitivity	Low Sensitivity
Lymphoid organs	Fine vasculature	Salivary glands
Bone marrow	Growing cartilage	Lungs
Testes	Growing bone	Kidneys
Intestines		Liver
		Optic lens

❏ **Radiosensitivity** is the difference in sensitivity of various cells and tissues. Some are more sensitive to the effects of ionizing radiation than others. The most sensitive cells are those which are rapidly reproducing, have a long mitotic period, and are poorly differentiated (Table 1-3).

❏ *Quality of the radiation* is another factor in determining biologic effect. Higher-energy radiations penetrate deeper and have a greater biologic effect than low-energy radiations.

❏ *Age at time of exposure* influences the harmful effects of radiation. Children are more sensitive to ionizing radiation than are adults. The embryo and fetus are particularly sensitive and should be exposed to radiation only in an emergency situation.

VI. PATIENT PROTECTION

The amount of ionizing radiation exposure during a dental examination is very small. However, any dose of ionizing radiation may cause biologic damage. It is important, therefore, that the operator use careful selection criteria and proper exposure and processing procedures for all patients.

A. National Guidelines

The following laws and guidelines for patient radiation protection have been established by various government agencies:

❏ **The ALARA Principle.** In 1954, the National Council on Radiation Protection (NCRP) put forth the principle that radiation exposures should be kept *as low as reasonably achievable* (ALARA). This concept recognizes that while there is a biologic effect from any dose of ionizing radiation, radiographs are necessary for complete patient assessment. It states that the patient should be exposed to the minimum amount of radiation required for adequate diagnosis and evaluation.

❏ **The Consumer–Patient Health and Safety Act of 1981.** This act requires that minimum education standards be set for all personnel who perform radiographic procedures. In order to expose radiographs on patients, dental hygienists and assistants must complete a recognized training program. Dental radiology courses in accredited dental hygiene and dental assisting programs are among those recognized.

❏ **Patient Selection Criteria.** In 1987, The U.S. Department of Health and Human Services published *The Selection of Patients for X-Ray Examinations: Dental Radiographic Examinations.* This document provides specific guidelines for exposing dental radiographs based on the patient's age, dental disease activity, and dentition. It is summarized in Table 1-4.

B. Clinical Recommendations

Radiographic Policies

All x-ray facilities should have written policies clearly stating the training requirements for x-ray personnel, patient selection criteria, and procedures for exposing radiographs and determining the need for retakes.

Patient Selection

The type and number of radiographs required for adequate patient assessment should be determined only after a review of the patient's medical and dental history and a complete clinical examination. Patients should never undergo routine x-ray examinations based solely on time intervals between exposures.

C. Equipment Factors

All x-ray equipment manufactured after 1974 must meet federal diagnostic equipment performance standards. Use of the equipment and inspection requirements are monitored by state and local agencies. Radiation equipment should be inspected at required intervals to ensure that it is functioning properly and that there is no radiation leakage. Some of the equipment factors that influence the patient's exposure to radiation are as follows:

❏ **Head leakage** is radiation leakage from the tube head. Since the tube head contains protective shielding designed to prevent radiation leakage, it is unlikely to occur unless the tube head is damaged. Head leakage unnecessarily exposes the patient to radiation. If the tube head has been moved, or if damage is suspected, the equipment should be examined and tested before it is used.

❏ **Drift** occurs when the tube head moves after it is positioned. It is caused by loose nuts and bolts in the adjusting arm that attaches the x-ray tube head to the wall. Tube drift may cause inaccurate radiographs and necessitate that films be retaken, creating an additional radiation exposure for the patient. The adjusting arm should be repaired immediately when drift occurs.

❏ **Filtration** removes long-wave x-ray photons which do not have sufficient energy to pass through structures and create the x-ray image. If these remained, they would cause an increase in the amount of radiation absorbed by the patient. Filtration is accomplished by placing aluminum disks in the path of the x-ray beam in the area where the beam exits the tube head (see Fig. 3-6). The aluminum filters absorb (attenuate) the unnecessary long-wave photons (see Chap. 3).

Table 1-4. Guidelines for Prescribing Radiographs

Patient Category	Child		Adolescent	Adult	
	Primary Dentition (*prior to eruption of first permanent tooth*)	Transitional Dentition (*following eruption of first permanent tooth*)	Permanent Dentition (*prior to eruption of third molars*)	Dentulous	Edentulous
New patient All new patients to assess dental diseases and growth and development	Posterior bitewing examination if proximal surfaces of primary teeth cannot be visualized or probed	Individualized radiographic examination consisting of periapical/occlusal views and posterior bitewings or panoramic examination and posterior bitewings	Individualized radiographic examination consisting of posterior bitewings and selected periapicals. A full-mouth intraoral radiographic examination is appropriate when the patient presents with clinical evidence of generalized dental disease or a history of extensive dental treatment.		Full mouth intraoral radiographic examination or panoramic examination
Recall patient Clinical caries or high-risk factors for caries	Posterior bitewing examination at 6-month intervals or until no carious lesions are evident	Posterior bitewing examination at 6-month intervals or until no carious lesions are evident	Posterior bitewing examination at 6- to 12-month intervals or until no carious lesions are evident	Posterior bitewing examination at 12- to 18-month intervals	Not applicable
No clinical caries and no high-risk factors for caries	Posterior bitewing examination at 12- to 24-month intervals if proximal surfaces of primary teeth cannot be visualized or probed	Posterior bitewing examination at 12- to 24-month intervals	Posterior bitewing examination at 18- to 36-month intervals	Posterior bitewing examination at 24- to 36-month intervals	Not applicable
Periodontal disease or a history of periodontal treatment	Individualized radiographic examination consisting of selected periapical and/or bitewing radiographs for areas where periodontal disease (other than nonspecific gingivitis) can be demonstrated clinically	Individualized radiographic examination consisting of selected periapical and/or bitewing radiographs for areas where periodontal disease (other than nonspecific gingivitis) can be demonstrated clinically	Individualized radiographic examination consisting of selected periapical and/or bitewing radiographs for areas where periodontal disease (other than nonspecific gingivitis) can be demonstrated clinically		Not applicable
Growth and development assessment	Usually not indicated	Individualized radiographic examination consisting of a periapical/occlusal or panoramic examination	Periapical or panoramic examination to assess developing third molars	Usually not indicated	Usually not indicated

❑ **Collimation** further reduces patient exposure to radiation by limiting the size of the area exposed. Collimation is accomplished by placing a flat lead disk with a small opening at its center in the path of the x-ray beam (see Fig. 3-7). This disk is called the *lead diaphragm* or *collimator.* The lead absorbs all the radiation that strikes it, while the opening allows radiation to pass through. The collimator is placed at the end of the position-indicating device which attaches to the x-ray machine (see Chap. 3).

❑ *Position-indicating devices (PIDs)* attach to the x-ray tube head and, if lead-lined, provide further collimation of the x-ray beam (see Fig. 3-3).

- The lead lining prevents radiation from passing through the PID, thereby limiting the size of the area exposed and eliminating scatter radiation that would occur if the x rays interacted with the PID.

- PIDs may be round or rectangular. The diameter of the x-ray beam at the end of a round, lead-lined PID is 2¾ in. The size of the x-ray beam at the end of a rectangular PID is 1¾ by 1⅝ in. Rectangular PIDs reduce the size of the area irradiated by 60 percent over round PIDs (Fig. 1-9).

- Older PIDs were not lead-lined. Some were short, plastic, pointed cones that were not open-ended. This type of PID should never be used because it provides no collimation of the x-ray beam, and scatter radiation is produced when x rays interact with the plastic.

❑ *Radiographic film* is the image receptor. Radiation chemically alters the film, creating the x-ray image (see Chap. 5). *Film speed* refers to the sensitivity of the film to radiation or the speed at which it reacts to radiation.

- X-ray film speeds range from A (slowest) to F (fastest) (see Chap. 3). Dental film is available in speeds D and E. E speed film is recommended because exposure time is 50 percent less than that of D speed film.

 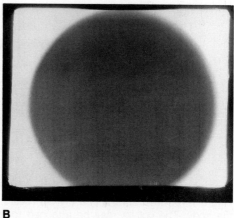

A   B

Figure 1-9. Rectangular PIDs **(A)** reduce the size of the area irradiated by 60 percent over round PIDs **(B)**.

- Radiographs exposed with E speed film may exhibit less sharpness and more fogging than those exposed with D speed film. The decrease in sharpness does not affect the diagnostic quality of the film. The quality of the image is improved with the use of rectangular collimation.

❏ The *timer* controls the duration of x-ray production and emission. The use of electronic timers is essential because old-fashioned mechanical timers cannot measure the extremely short exposure times required by fast-speed films. The accuracy of the timers should be checked at regular intervals.

❏ *Aiming devices* are available to assist the operator in the correct alignment of the film and radiation beam to the teeth (see Chap. 3). Because the use of aiming devices significantly reduces film retakes caused by errors in technique, they should be used whenever possible.

❏ *Lead aprons and thyroid collars* should be used for all exposures and should cover the patient from the thyroid to the gonadal area (Fig. 1-10). The aprons and collars may contain a thin layer of lead or be constructed from lead-impregnated plastic. They prevent primary radi-

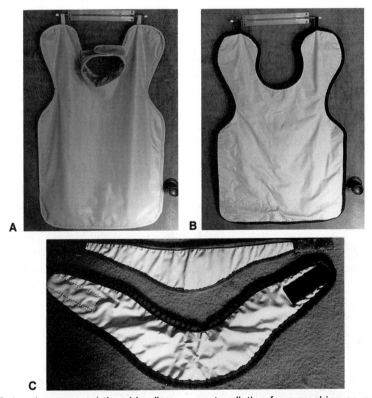

Figure 1-10. Lead aprons and thyroid collars prevent radiation from reaching covered parts of the body. The collars may be attached to the apron **(A)** or used separated from the apron **(B)**. They are also available in a children's size **(C**, at top).

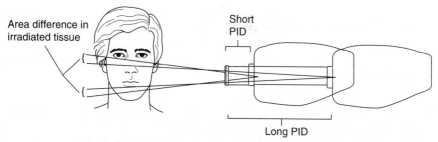

Figure 1-11. The use of a long PID reduces the amount of tissue irradiated because the radiation beam diverges less as the distance from the radiation source increases.

ation from reaching the covered parts of the body. Lead aprons are available in child and adult sizes with or without attached thyroid collars. Separate thyroid collars are available. The lead-lined aprons and collars should not be folded. This may cause the lead to crack, reducing their effectiveness. When not in use, aprons may be hung on hangers, available from manufacturers of dental x-ray supplies.

D. Technique Factors

It is important that the operator pay careful attention to exposure and processing techniques to produce diagnostically acceptable radiographs. Unacceptable radiographs necessitate that films be retaken, exposing the patient to additional ionizing radiation. The following are important technique considerations:

❒ The *parallel technique* (see Chap. 8) is preferred because the resulting radiograph more accurately represents the size, shape, and location of structures. The use of a long PID reduces the amount of tissue irradiated because the radiation beam diverges less as the distance from the radiation source increases (Fig. 1-11). In addition, there is less exposure to the sensitive tissues of the thyroid and eye lens because of the small angulation of the radiation beam with this technique.

❒ *Processing procedures* (see Chap. 5) must be followed carefully whether manual or automatic processing is used. Proper maintenance of the darkroom, its solutions, and equipment is essential. Patient films must be labeled accurately and filed. Unexposed films should be stored at 50 to 70°F to prevent deterioration. Expiration dates should be monitored. Darkroom errors and improper film handling can necessitate retakes of films which would otherwise have been adequate.

SUMMARY RECOMMENDATIONS FOR PATIENT PROTECTION

To summarize the preceding concepts, it is recommended that the following steps be taken to ensure that patient exposure to ionizing radiation is *as low as* reasonably *a*chievable:

- Establish a regular schedule for equipment monitoring and maintenance.
- Training must be provided to all personnel who are responsible for exposing radiographs.
- Review the patient's medical and dental histories, perform a clinical examination, and use patient selection criteria when determining the need for radiographs.
- Use rectangular PIDs with aiming devices.
- Use E speed film.
- Use a lead apron and thyroid collar for all exposures.
- Expose radiographs using the parallel technique and a 16-in PID whenever possible.
- Take care in film handling and processing, and monitor and maintain darkroom equipment and solutions.

VII. OPERATOR PROTECTION

Any exposure to ionizing radiation can cause damage to the operator as well as the patient. The ALARA concept must be followed for both. Dental radiographers should strive for zero exposure even though federal standards may make it appear that some exposure is acceptable or inevitable. **Maximum permissible dose (MPD)** is the maximum dose of whole-body radiation that the federal government allows radiation workers to receive. It is currently 0.05 Sv (5 rem) per year. This is 10 times the MPD for the general population.

Careful adherence to radiation hygiene procedures will eliminate the risk of exposure.

A. Barriers

In order to protect the operator and other personnel from exposure, a barrier must be in place. Various types of barriers are used.

Free-standing barriers will protect the operator but will not protect other personnel or patients in some settings. Walls, ceilings, and floors must be constructed using material of sufficient density to absorb primary and secondary radiation. The National Committee on Radiation Protection (NCRP) Report No. 35 provides specifications for construction materials that will provide shielding in specific situations. Lead-lined doors with a contact that prevents the x-ray machine from operating unless the door is closed provide an excellent barrier when combined with adequately lined walls.

B. Positioning

The position of the operator in relation to the x-ray beam can play an important role in reducing radiation exposure. If an adequate barrier is unavailable, the operator should stand a minimum of 6 ft from the patient at an angle of from 90 to 135 degrees to the primary beam of radiation.

C. Exposure Technique

Radiation exposure to the operator as well as the patient can be reduced by using proper exposure technique. The operator should never hold the film for the patient. If the patient is unable to hold the film, even with the aid of holders, a member of the patient's family should assist. The operator must never stabilize the tube head by holding it. A drifting tube head must be repaired before further exposures are made.

D. Monitoring

Radiation exposure to personnel may be monitored through the use of a film badge. This is a radiosensitive material encased in plastic that can be clipped to clothing while in the radiography area. Monitoring companies provide and periodically collect film badges to measure radiation exposure. The company then submits a written report of the individual occupational exposure for all personnel monitored.

SUMMARY RECOMMENDATIONS FOR OPERATOR PROTECTION

- Follow the ALARA concept, and strive for zero occupational exposures.
- Make all exposures behind adequate barriers.
- Never hold the film or tube head during exposures.
- Protect other personnel and patients from inadvertent exposure with appropriate barriers.
- Monitor radiation exposure.

REVIEW EXERCISES

1. In the space provided below, draw an oxygen atom. Label the nucleus, energy shells, electrons, protons, and neutrons.

2. Define *binding energy.*

3. In the space provided, draw a water molecule. Label the nuclei, energy shells, protons, neutrons, and electrons.

4. Define *ionization*, and draw a diagram of it.

5. In the space provided, list eight types of electromagnetic radiation. What characteristics do they have in common? Which has the most energy? Why?

6. In the space provided, list and describe three results of the interaction of x rays with matter:

7. List and give examples of three types of biologic damage which may result from exposure to ionizing radiation.

8. List and explain six factors which influence the biologic effects of radiation.

9. List three factors which influence cell radiosensitivity.

10. List six cells or tissues which are highly radiosensitive.

11. Define the ALARA principle.

12. Describe the patient protection provided by the Consumer Health and Safety Act of 1981.

13. Describe the influence of the following equipment factors on radiation protection.

    Head leakage

    Tube head drift

    Filtration

    Collimation

    Film

    Timer

    Aiming devices

    Lead aprons and thyroid collars

14. Describe the influence of the following technique factors on radiation protection.

    The parallel technique

    16-in PID

    Processing techniques and procedures

15. Describe the influence of the following on radiation protection for the operator.

MPD

Barriers

Positioning

Exposure technique

Monitoring

16. Define all the terms listed at the end of the Learning Objectives in this chapter.

LEARNING ACTIVITIES

Learning Activity 1-1: Exposure and Dose

Equipment:

1 kitchen sponge
1 bowl or other container for the sponge
1 beaker or other liquid measure with measurements to 16 oz

Activity:

1. Place the sponge in the container.
2. Fill beaker with water to the 16-oz mark.
3. Pour the water on the sponge, allowing a minute for the sponge to absorb the water.
4. Remove the sponge, and pour the water remaining in the container into the beaker.
5. Record the number of ounces remaining: _____.

Questions:

1. In ounces, to how much water was the sponge exposed?

   _____

2. In ounces, how much water did the sponge absorb?

   _____

3. Relate this to exposure and dose in radiology.

Learning Activity 1-2: Facility Assessment

Equipment:

None

Activity:

Evaluate your dental radiology facility based on the information and criteria in this chapter. What can be done to improve radiation protection?

Strengths: **Weaknesses:**

Recommendations:

Learning Activity 1-3: Patient Selection

do for 3/25

Equipment:

None

Activity:

Use the patient selection criteria provided in this chapter to determine the type and number of radiographs (if any) required in the following situations.

Case 1

It is the first dental visit for a 4-year-old. The primary dentition is present and normal. The contacts between the primary

Recommended Radiographs:

None because no caries + all surfaces

Why? *can be examined visually.*

molars are open. No clinical signs of disease or carious lesions are present. Permanent teeth are unerupted.

Case 2

This is the first visit to this office for a healthy 42-year-old woman. Her last dental radiographs were bitewings taken 3 years ago at her last dental visit. At that time, both mandibular first molars were abscessed and extracted. All other teeth are present. There are numerous large amalgam restorations. The gingiva is inflamed, and 4- to 6-mm pockets are generalized.

Recommended Radiographs:

FMX to assess disease and because of extensive previous dental work

Why?

Case 3

Your patient is an 8-year-old girl. None of the permanent teeth have yet erupted. Carious lesions are present on the occlusal surfaces of A, J, and S.

Recommended Radiographs:

post BW, & selected PA.

Why? *because of caries & the fact no perm. teeth yet erupted.*

Case 4

A 53-year-old man whose last dental examination was 6 months ago is your patient. Bitewing radiographs were taken 1 year ago and show no evidence of caries or periodontal disease. At this visit, no carious lesions or symptoms of periodontal disease are detected.

Recommended Radiographs:

none

Why? *no caries & recommended interval is 24-36 mo*

BIBLIOGRAPHY

De Lyre, W. R., and Johnson, O. N. *Essentials of Dental Radiology for Dental Assistants and Hygienists,* 4th ed. Norwalk, Conn., Appleton and Lange, 1990.

Goaz, P. W., and White, S. C. *Oral Radiology.* St. Louis, C.V. Mosby, 1987.

Frommer, H. H. *Radiology for Dental Auxiliaries,* 5th ed. St. Louis, Mosby–Year Book, 1992.

U.S. Department of Health and Human Services, Public Health Service, FDA. *The Selection of Patients for X-Ray Examinations, Dental Radiographic Examinations* (HSS/PHS/FDA 88-8273). Washington, U.S. Government Printing Office, 1987, pp. 10–21.

Infection Control

2

After completing this chapter the student will be able to

1. Describe the rationale for infection control in dental radiographic procedures.
2. Describe and demonstrate barriers to infection, including
   Operator attire
   Equipment barriers/wraps
3. Describe and demonstrate appropriate infection-control procedures when preparing the operatory for a patient.
4. Describe and demonstrate appropriate infection-control procedures for exposing radiographs on patients.
5. Describe and demonstrate appropriate infection-control procedures in manual and automatic processing.

Each dental radiography facility varies in design and use. Infection-control protocols must be designed to meet the specific needs of each facility. This chapter describes general infection-control guidelines for dental radiography procedures which may be adapted to the design, use, and procedures in your facility.

I. INFECTION-CONTROL PROCEDURES

Any dental practitioner or patient may harbor pathogenic microorganisms which may be transmitted to others. The human immunodeficiency virus (HIV) is present in saliva and may be transmitted by contact with the infected person's blood. Hepatitis may be transmitted by contact with infected blood or saliva. Infections with resistant strains of tuberculosis are increasing and are transmitted by airborne microorganisms. These are only a few of the many infectious diseases which may be spread from person to person in the absence of infection-control procedures.

During oral radiographic procedures, the operator is in close contact with the patient and must touch several surfaces after placing films in the oral cavity, where saliva and possibly blood are present. Proper infection-control procedures are necessary to prevent disease transmission from operator to patient, patient to operator, or patient to patient or other office personnel.

A. Preparation of the Operatory

All surfaces that will come in contact with the patient or operator during the appointment should be disinfected with an Environmental Protection Agency (EPA)–registered American Dental Association (ADA)–approved surface disinfectant and/or covered *before* seating the patient (Fig. 2-1).

❑ Disinfect
- Chair and headrest
- Chair controls
- PID, tube head, and yoke
- Doorknobs
- Control panel
- Activating button
- Faucets, handles, and soap dispensers (foot controls preferred)
- Any other surfaces touched during the appointment

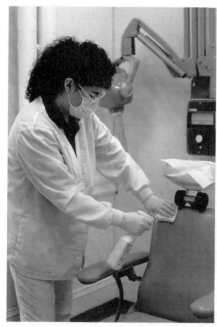
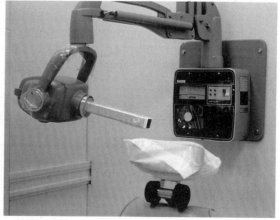

A   **B**

Figure 2-1. Surface disinfection. All surfaces that come in contact with the patient or operator during the appointment should be **(A)** disinfected and/or **(B)** covered before seating the patient.

❏ Cover
- Headrest
- Chair controls
- Control panel
- Activating button
- PID (Do not cover open end. This will create scattered radiation.)
- Tube head and yoke
- Doorknobs

B. Routine Cleaning and Maintenance

❏ Clean sinks, counters, and equipment regularly.

❏ Dispose of trash following local, Occupational Safety and Health Administration (OSHA), and EPA regulations.

C. Appointment Procedures for Infection Control

Treat all patients as though they were infectious.

❏ A complete medical history must be taken and reviewed on all patients. (While this may alert the operator to medical conditions that require special consideration, many infectious patients will not be identified by their medical history.)

❏ Keep patient records away from any source of contamination.

❏ The operator must wear eyeglasses with sideshields, a mask, gloves, and attire that meets OSHA regulations during the appointment (Fig. 2-2).

❏ Wash hands before and after wearing gloves.

❏ Wear gloves whenever handling contaminated film packets, supplies, and aiming devices and during cleanup procedures.

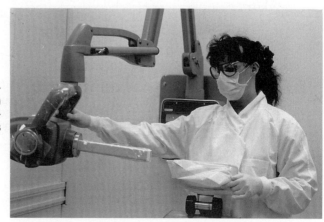

Figure 2-2. Operator attire. The operator must wear eyeglasses with sideshields, a mask, gloves, and attire that meets OSHA regulations during the appointment.

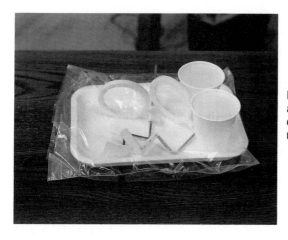

Figure 2-3. Sample tray setup, with aiming devices, a cup containing required films, and a cup for contaminated films.

☐ If possible, determine the type, number, and size of films required prior to seating the patient. Wear clean gloves to place the required films, aiming devices, and other supplies on a disinfected, covered tray (Fig. 2-3). Barrier envelopes are available to protect film packets from contamination (Fig. 2-4). If these are used, the films should be placed in the envelopes at this time.

☐ Disinfect and cover work surfaces prior to seating the patient (see Fig. 2-1).

☐ Place contaminated films in a disposable cup (see Fig. 2-3).

☐ Sterilize all instruments and equipment that come in contact with blood and/or saliva with heat or gas. Where this is impossible, chemical disinfection may be used with appropriate contact times.

☐ Wear gloves during cleanup. Contaminated gloves may be worn to remove covers and wraps and to discard disposables. Remove contaminated gloves, wash hands, and put on new gloves before disinfecting and covering for the next patient.

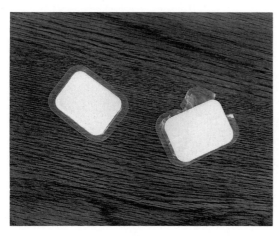

Figure 2-4. Barrier envelopes may be used to protect the films from contamination.

❏ Discard contaminated gloves and masks and wash hands before leaving the radiography area. OSHA guidelines must be followed for the removal and laundering of attire.

D. Preparation of the Darkroom and Processing

❏ Disinfect and/or cover all surfaces that contact contaminated films or gloves prior to each use. If possible, the darkroom should be prepared for processing when the operatory is prepared.

❏ Wear gloves when handling contaminated films or touching contaminated surfaces.

❏ Cover an area on the counter on which to place the cup with the contaminated films.

❏ Place a clean cup or paper towel on the disinfected counter for unwrapped films.

❏ When entering the darkroom, doors and other surfaces should not be contaminated.

❏ Take care not to touch the film packet with contaminated gloves when removing barrier envelopes (Fig. 2-5). Pull the envelope apart and drop the films onto the clean towel or into a clean paper cup. Remove contaminated gloves, wash hands, and proceed with processing (see Chap. 5).

❏ Wear gloves to unwrap films not encased in barrier envelopes (Fig. 2-6). Under safelight conditions, pull the plastic film wrapper apart, being careful not to touch the inner contents, and drop the contents onto the clean towel or into the clean paper cup. Remove contaminated gloves, wash hands, and proceed with processing.

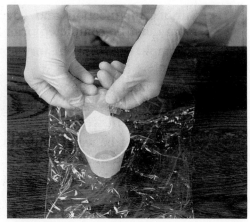

Figure 2-5. Unwrapping film-barrier envelope. Being careful not to touch the film, pull the envelope apart, and drop the film onto a covered work surface or into a clean paper cup.

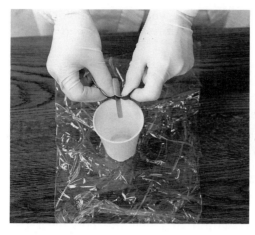

Figure 2-6. Unwrapping film packet. Being careful not to touch the inner film components, pull the wrapper apart, and drop the components onto a covered work surface or into a clean paper cup.

Note: Contamination is difficult to avoid with the use of daylight loaders unless barrier envelopes are used and removed prior to processing.

II. IMMUNIZATIONS

Since dental workers are at risk for contracting the hepatitis B virus, immunization against this virus is highly recommended. Other recommended immunizations should be current.

SUMMARY OF INFECTION-CONTROL RECOMMENDATIONS

- A written infection-control policy should be in place for all dental facilities.
- A dental professional should have the responsibility for developing, implementing, and monitoring infection-control policies and practices in the facility.
- Surface disinfection and covering in the operatory and darkroom must be completed prior to seating the patient.
- A complete medical history should be taken and reviewed on all patients.
- Hands must be washed before and after wearing gloves.
- Gloves, masks, and eyeglasses with sideshields must be worn during patient treatment.
- Gloves must be worn while handling contaminated film packets, supplies, and instruments.
- Gloves must be worn during cleanup and disinfection procedures.

- All surfaces touched during the appointment must be disinfected and/or covered.
- Whenever possible, the size, type, and number of films should be determined and dispensed prior to seating the patient.
- All equipment and instruments that come in contact with blood, saliva, or contaminated films should be sterilized. Where this is impossible and on surfaces, chemical disinfectants may be used with proper contact time.
- Remove contaminated gloves and attire and wash hands before leaving the treatment area.
- Follow OSHA guidelines.

REVIEW EXERCISES

1. Describe the rationale for infection control in radiography procedures.

inf can be spread via saliva &/or blood, and transferred from person to person (pt and/or operator) manually or on contaminated equipment.

2. List the surfaces that must be disinfected prior to seating the patient.

chair, headrest, controls, PID, Tubehead & yoke, doorknobs, cont panel, exp button, faucets, handles, soap dispensors

3. List those surfaces which must be covered during an appointment.

Headrest, Chair controls, Cont panel, exp butt, PID Except open end.

4. Describe infection-control procedures for radiography appointments.

Med Hx, keep pt records away from source of contam. Wear eyeglasses, mask, gloves, & proper attire

5. Describe appropriate infection-control procedures for manual and automatic processing.

Wear glo handling contaminated films or touching cont. surfaces. Do not touch film packet c contam glo when removing protective env, then remove gloves. If no prot env used, then wear glo. to unwrap films.

LEARNING ACTIVITIES

Learning Activity 2-1: Facility Assessment

Equipment:

None

Activity:

Assess the infection-control practices at your facility.

Strengths: **Weaknesses:**

Recommendations:

Learning Activity 2-2: Infection-Control Procedures

Equipment:

    Surface disinfectant
    Covering material
    Eyeglasses with sideshields
    1 mask
    Gloves
    1 clean paper cup or paper towel
    1 film packet

Locations:

    The x-ray operatory
    The darkroom

Activity:

1. Following recommended procedures, prepare the radiography operatory for patient treatment by disinfecting and covering appropriate surfaces.

2. Demonstrate correct operator attire.

3. Demonstrate correct disinfection and covering of darkroom surfaces.

4. Unwrap a film without contaminating the contents.

BIBLIOGRAPHY

Proposed infection control guidelines for dental radiographic procedures. *American Academy of Oral and Maxillofacial Radiology Newsletter* 17(1):10–11, 1990.

Frommer, H. H. *Radiology for Dental Auxiliaries,* 5th ed. St. Louis, Mosby–Year Book, 1992.

Equipment and the Production of X Rays

3

After completing this chapter the student will be able to

1. Identify the following parts of the dental x-ray machine, and describe and demonstrate the function of each:

   X-ray tube head

   Adjusting arm

   Position indicating devices (PIDs)

   Control panel—mA, ammeter, kVp, voltmeter, timer, on/off switch

   Activating button

   Aluminum filter

   Lead diaphragm

   Number scale

2. Make adjustments in:

   Exposure time

   Milliamperage (mA)

   Kilovolt peak (kVp)

   Vertical and horizontal angulation

3. Calculate mAs (milliampere-seconds) and exposure time or mA (milliamperes) required to achieve a given mAs level.

4. Convert exposure time from impulses to seconds and from seconds to impulses.

5. Label the parts of the x-ray tube, and describe their function.

6. Describe the components of the anode–cathode and filament circuits, and describe their function.

7. Describe the production of x rays.

8. Describe adjustments which influence x-ray quality and quantity.

9. State and explain the inverse-square law.

10. Identify the following dental film sizes, and describe their recommended uses:

0

1

2

3

4

11. Identify the following components of x-ray film, and describe the purpose of each:

Base

Emulsion

Lead foil

Black paper

Plastic wrapper/color-coded tab

12. Identify and assemble the following film holders/aiming devices, and describe the advantages and disadvantages of each:

Stabe film holder

Rinn XCP instrument

Rinn BAI instrument

Precision instrument

13. Define the following terms:

Amperage (ampere, milliampere)

Bremsstrahlung x rays

Collimation

Current

Film density

Film speed

Filtration

Focal spot (actual, effective)

Half-value layer (HVL)

Horizontal angulation

Intensity of the x-ray beam

Rectification (self)

Scale of contrast (long, short)

Thermionic emission

Transformer

Tube–film distance (TFD)

Vertical angulation (positive, negative)

Voltage (volt, kilovolt)

I. THE X-RAY MACHINE

A. The X-Ray Tube Head

The x-ray tube that produces the x-ray beam is contained in the *x-ray tube head.* It is attached to the wall by the *adjusting arm* which allows

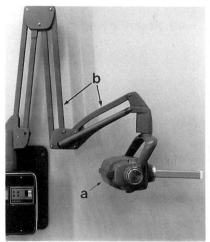
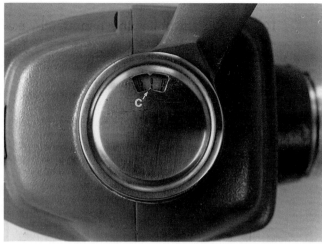

Figure 3-1. The x-ray tube head. (a) The tube head. (b) The adjusting arm. (c) The number scale at the side of the tube head indicates the degree of vertical angulation in use.

large movements of the tube head (Fig. 3-1). The tube head may be rotated from side to side in a horizontal plane to make adjustments in the **horizontal angulation** of the x-ray beam (Fig. 3-2A). It also may be tilted up and down in a vertical plane to make adjustments in **vertical angulation** (Fig. 3-2B). If the x-ray beam is directed toward the floor, **positive vertical angulation** is in use. If it is directed toward the ceiling, **negative vertical angulation** is in use.

B. The Number Scale

Located on the side of the tube head, the *number scale* identifies the degree of vertical angulation in use (Fig. 3-1, right). If the x-ray beam is directed downward and the number scale on the side of the tube indicates 20, the angulation is 20 degrees positive (20+). If it is directed upward and the scale indicates 20, the angulation is 20 degrees negative (20−).

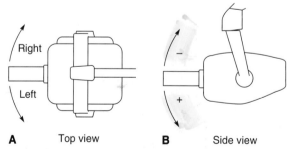

Figure 3-2. **(A)** Movement of the x-ray tube head from left to right in a horizontal plane allows adjustments in horizontal angulation. **(B)** Movement of the x-ray tube head up or down in a vertical plane adjusts the vertical angulation of the x-ray beam. If the PID is directed downward, the vertical angulation is positive. If it is directed upward, the vertical angulation is negative.

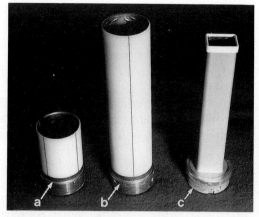

Figure 3-3. PIDs. (a) A short, round PID. (b) A long, round PID. (c) A long, rectangular PID. All are open-ended and lead-lined.

When not in use, the tube head should be positioned against the wall with the *position-indicating device* (PID) directed at the floor.

C. The Position-Indicating Device (PID)

The *position-indicating device (PID)* is attached to the x-ray tube head and assists in aiming the x-ray beam. PIDs may be round or rectangular and should be lead-lined and open-ended. PIDs are classified as short, intermediate, or long, with lengths varying according to the manufacturers tube-head design (Fig. 3-3).

D. The Control Panel

The controls for the x-ray machine are located on the *control panel* (Fig. 3-4). Its location and design vary by manufacturer. The following will be found on most control panels:

❏ The *on/off switch* turns the machine on and off and may control a light which, when lit, indicates that the machine is turned on. When not in use, the machine should be turned off.

❏ The *kilovolt peak (kVp) selector* determines the peak voltage at which

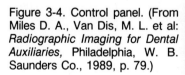

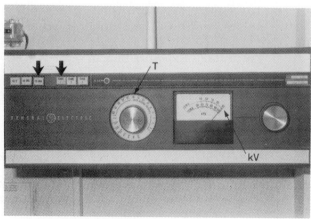

Figure 3-4. Control panel. (From Miles D. A., Van Dis, M. L. et al: *Radiographic Imaging for Dental Auxiliaries,* Philadelphia, W. B. Saunders Co., 1989, p. 79.)

the machine operates. Most dental x-ray machines are operated at settings of 65 to 90 kVp. As the setting increases, the *penetrating power* of the x-ray beam increases.

❏ The *voltmeter* measures and indicates kilovolts during each exposure.

❏ The *milliamperage (mA) control* determines the *amount* of radiation produced during each exposure. Dental x-ray machines operate at either 10 or 15 mA. More radiation is produced at 15 mA than at 10 mA.

❏ The *timer* determines the *duration* of radiation production. X rays are produced in $\frac{1}{120}$-s impulses rather than in a constant stream. For this reason, modern x-ray machines measure exposure time in impulses rather than seconds. With 60-cycle alternating current, there are 60 impulses of x rays each second. A setting of 6 impulses equals a $\frac{1}{10}$-s setting; 30 impulses equals a $\frac{1}{2}$-s exposure.

EXPOSURE TIME CONVERSIONS

- To convert exposure time in impulses to exposure time in seconds, *divide* the number of impulses by 60.

Formula: $\dfrac{\text{Number of impulses}}{60}$ = exposure time in seconds

Example: 6 impulses = __?__ seconds

Solution: $\frac{6}{60}$ = $\frac{1}{10}$ second

Example: 30 impulses = __?__ seconds

Solution: $\frac{30}{60}$ = $\frac{1}{2}$ second

- To convert exposure time in seconds to exposure time in impulses, *multiply* the number of seconds by 60.

Formula: Exposure time in seconds × 60 = exposure time in impulses

Example: $\frac{1}{5}$ second = __?__ impulses

Solution: $\frac{1}{5}$ × 60 = $\frac{60}{5}$ = 12 impulses

Example: $\frac{1}{4}$ second = __?__ impulses

Solution: $\frac{1}{4}$ × 60 = $\frac{60}{4}$ = 15 impulses

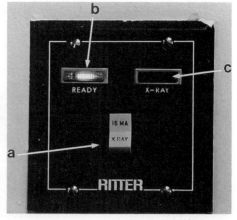

Figure 3-5. This activating button (a) is mounted on a lead-lined wall. When it is depressed, x rays are emitted from the machine. It has an indicator light (b) that is lit when the machine is on and an indicator light (c) that flashes during the exposure.

E. The Activating Button

The *activating button* may be located at the end of a cord, in a foot pedal, or mounted in a lead-lined wall outside the x-ray room (Fig. 3-5). Whatever the type of activating button, it must allow the operator to stand a minimum of 6 ft away from the patient and behind an effective radiation barrier.

F. The Aluminum Filter

The *aluminum filter* is an aluminum disk placed in the path of the x-ray beam to absorb low-energy x rays that do not have the penetrating power to pass through anatomic structures and reach the film (Fig. 3-6). Without this **filtration,** these x rays would remain and cause an increase in the amount of radiation absorbed by the patient (see Chap. 1). Federal regulations require that the disks be 1.5 mm thick if the machine is operated below 70 kVp and 2.5 mm thick if it is operated above 70 kVp.

G. The Lead Diaphragm or Collimator

Collimation further reduces patient exposure to radiation by limiting the size of the area exposed. The device which collimates the x-ray beam in

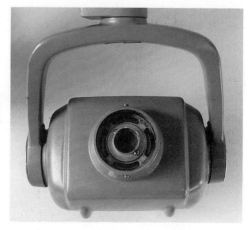

Figure 3-6. The aluminum filter is placed in the path of the x-ray beam where it exits the tube head. It removes nonuseful low-energy x rays from the beam.

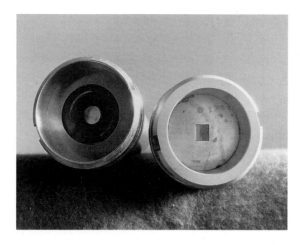

Figure 3-7. Lead collimators are placed at the end of the PID that attaches to the tube head. They restrict the size of the x-ray beam.

dental x-ray machines is the *lead diaphragm,* a flat lead disk with a small opening at its center through which radiation passes. It is located at the end of the PID that attaches to the tube head. It may be round or rectangular depending on the shape of the PID in use (Fig. 3-7). Lead-lined PIDs provide further **collimation** to the x-ray beam after it passes through the lead diaphragm (see Chap. 1).

II. PRODUCTION OF THE X-RAY BEAM

A. The X-Ray Tube

Within the x-ray tube head is a vacuum tube containing the components that produce the x-ray beam (Fig. 3-8).

- ☐ The *cathode* is the negative electrode. Electrons are produced at the cathode and used in the production of x rays. The cathode consists of two primary parts:
  - The *tungsten filament* is a thin, coiled tungsten wire mounted on two strong wires which support it and provide electricity. Electrons emitted from the filament are used in the production of x rays.

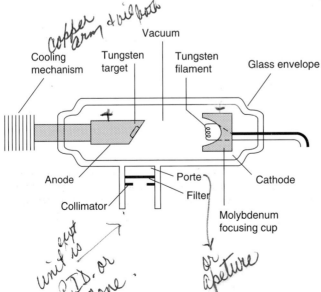

Figure 3-8. The dental x-ray tube and its components.

- The *molybdenum focusing cup* contains the tungsten filament and focuses its electrons into a narrow beam directed at the focal spot or target located on the anode.

❏ The *anode* is the positive electrode. The energy of the electrons produced by the cathode are converted to x-ray and heat energy when they strike the target in the anode. The anode is composed of two primary parts:

- The *tungsten target* is the area on the anode that the electrons strike. The target converts the kinetic energy of the electrons into x-ray energy. This is a very inefficient process; less than 1 percent of the kinetic energy is converted to x rays, and the rest becomes heat. Tungsten is the target material of choice because of its high melting point and low vapor pressure at high temperatures. Because tungsten has a high atomic number and high density, it is very efficient at producing x rays.

- The *copper stem* contains the tungsten target. Because tungsten is a poor heat conductor, the tungsten target is embedded in the copper stem. Copper is an excellent heat conductor and dissipates the heat from the tube into the tube head, where it is cooled by air or oil immersion.

B. Electrical Wiring

The dental x-ray machine operates on 60-cycle 110-V alternating current.

❏ **Current** is the flow of electricity through a circuit. *Alternating current* flows in one direction to a peak voltage and then in the opposite direction. The flow of electricity in one direction and then the opposite is a *cycle* (Fig. 3-9). There are 60 cycles each second.

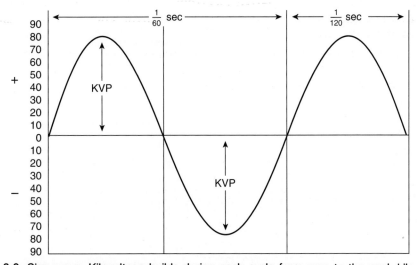

Figure 3-9. Sine wave. Kilovoltage builds during each cycle from zero to the peak kilovoltage determined by the kilovoltage setting. It then returns to zero before the current reverses direction. X rays are produced for half of each cycle (¹⁄₁₂₀ second). During the second half of the cycle, the current reverses direction and the polarity of the electrodes changes. At this time, no x rays are produced.

❏ **Voltage** is the electrical *force* that pushes the electricity through the circuit. It is measured in **volts.** A **kilovolt** is 1000 volts.

❏ **Amperage** is the *amount* of electricity in a circuit. It is measured in **amperes** *(amps).* A **milliampere** is 1/1000 amps.

❏ A **transformer** is a device used to increase or decrease the voltage in a circuit.

Electric circuits. There are two electric circuits in the dental x-ray machine (Fig. 3-10):

❏ The *anode–cathode circuit* or *high-voltage circuit* provides the electric charge to the anode (+) and cathode (−). It requires 65,000 to 90,000 V (65 to 90 kVp). The following components are included in the anode–cathode circuit:

   • The *step-up transformer* is used to increase the line voltage to the required 65,000 to 90,000 V.
   • The *kilovolt peak (kVp) selector.*
   • The *voltmeter.*
   • The *activating button.*
   • The *timer.*
   • The *x-ray emission light* and/or *sound.*

❏ The *filament circuit* provides electricity to the tungsten filament in the cathode. This circuit requires only 3 to 5 V. The following components are included in the filament circuit:

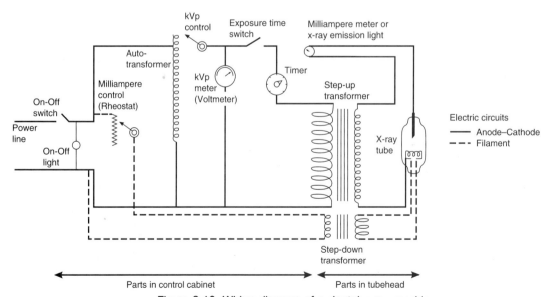

Figure 3-10. Wiring diagram of a dental x-ray machine.

- The *step-down transformer* reduces the line voltage from 110 to 3 to 5 V.
- The *on/off switch* and *light*.
- The *milliamperage (mA) control*.

C. Production of X-Rays

1. X rays are produced in the tube head in the following sequence (Fig. 3-11): When the x-ray machine is turned on, electricity flows through the filament circuit, heating the tungsten filament.
   Note: The amount of electricity flowing through the circuit is controlled by the milliamperage control knob. Dental x-ray machines operate at either 10 or 15 mA. At 15 mA, more current flows through the circuit than at 10 mA, and the filament becomes hotter.

2. When the filament is heated, it emits electrons by **thermionic emission.** Emitted electrons are replaced because the negative side of the high-voltage circuit is connected to one of the filament mounting wires. The emitted electrons form a cloud around the filament.
   Note: At higher filament temperatures, more electrons are emitted. If there are more electrons, more x rays will be produced. Therefore, milliamperage controls the temperature of the filament, the number of electrons emitted, and the number of x rays produced.

3. When the activating button is pushed, the anode–cathode circuit is activated and the anode (+) and cathode (−) are charged. The amount of charge is controlled by the kilovoltage setting.

4. The negatively charged electrons are repelled from the cathode (−) and travel at high speeds across the x-ray tube.

5. The molybdenum focusing cup directs the electrons in a narrow beam at the focal spot or target located on the anode.

6. When the electrons strike the anode (+) at the tungsten target, their kinetic energy is transformed into heat and x-ray energy.

Figure 3-11. X-ray production. When the activating button is pressed, the electrodes are charged, and the cloud of electrons created at the tungsten filament travel across the tube, striking the tungsten target. X-ray and heat energy are produced.

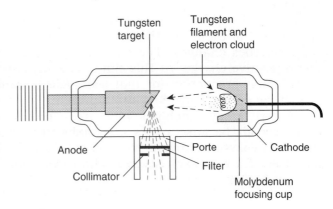

Note: The amount of charge to the anode and cathode is controlled by the kilovoltage setting. At higher settings, the charge is greater. The electrons travel at higher speeds and strike the target with more force, creating more powerful x rays with shorter wavelengths.

7. The angle of the target projects the x rays out of the tube through a thinner area of glass called the *porte.* The x-ray tube head is lead-lined, preventing x rays from exiting the tube head at any point except the porte.
   Note: The tungsten target is angled to project a smaller **effective focal spot** than the **actual focal spot** (the target) where the x rays are produced. This enhances the sharpness of the radiographic image and allows the heat generated by x-ray production to be dissipated over a large area.

8. The aluminum filter removes low-energy x rays from the x-ray beam.

9. The lead diaphragm and PID collimate the x-ray beam, reducing the area exposed to radiation.

Most of the x rays created are **Bremsstrahlung (braking) x rays.** These x rays are created when the high-speed electrons strike the target and interact with the tungsten atoms. An electron may hit a nucleus and have all its energy converted to a single x-ray photon, or it may be attracted toward a positively charged nucleus and diverted from its path. As it changes direction, some of its kinetic energy is converted to x-ray energy. The closer the electron is to the nucleus, the greater will be the energy of the resultant x-ray photon. Bremsstrahlung x rays have varying wavelengths and energies.

Because most dental x-ray machines use alternating current, the kilovoltage builds during each cycle from zero to the peak kilovoltage determined by the kilovoltage setting. It then returns to zero before the current reverses direction. X rays produced at a higher kilovoltage will have shorter wavelengths and more energy than those produced at a lower kilovoltage. The x-ray beam is said to be *heterogeneous* because it consists of x-ray photons of varying wavelengths produced by differing kilovoltages.

X rays are produced for half of each cycle ($\frac{1}{120}$ second). During the second half of the cycle, the current reverses direction, and the polarity of the electrodes changes. The electrons remain at the cathode, which now has a positive charge. At this time, no x rays are produced. This blocking of radiation production for half the cycle is caused by the design of the x-ray tube and is called **self-rectification.**

Modern x-ray machines measure exposure time in impulses rather than seconds because x rays are produced in $\frac{1}{120}$-second impulses rather than in a constant stream. With 60-cycle alternating current, there are 60 impulses of x rays each second. The timer controls the duration of radiation production.

D. Adjustments that Influence X-Ray Quality and Quantity

The *quality* or penetrating power of the x-ray beam is controlled by the kilovoltage setting. The x-ray beam must have sufficient power to demonstrate the different densities of objects on film. It should pass through less dense objects while it is increasingly absorbed by objects of increasing density. At higher kilovoltage settings, the x-ray beam has more penetrating power. Settings from 65 to 90 kVp are used in dental radiography.

❑ Dental radiographs are black-and-white images of dental structures. The varying shades of gray in the images demonstrate the **scale of contrast** of the film (Fig. 3-12). Films exposed at lower kilovoltage settings do not demonstrate many variations in radiation absorption. They exhibit fewer shades of gray and therefore have a **short scale of contrast.** Films exposed at higher kilovoltage settings demonstrate many variations in radiation absorption by structures. They exhibit many shades of gray and have a **long scale of contrast.**

❑ **Half-value layer (HVL)** is the measurement of the quality of the x rays emitted from an x-ray machine. It is the thickness in millimeters of aluminum that will reduce the intensity of an x-ray beam by 50 percent. An x-ray beam with a half-value layer of 4 has more penetrating power than one with an HVL of 3.

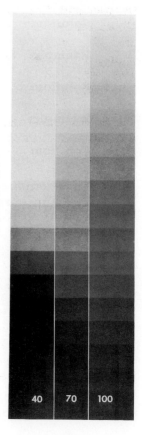

Figure 3-12. Scale of contrast appears in the radiograph as gradations in shades of gray from black to white. A short scale of contrast (high contrast) occurs when the film exhibits very black areas and white areas with few shades of gray *(left band).* A long scale of contrast (low contrast) occurs when the film exhibits many shades of gray as well as black and white *(right band).* The scale of contrast in a radiograph increases as the kilovoltage increases. (From Miles D. A., Van Dis, M. L. et al: *Radiographic Imaging for Dental Auxiliaries,* 2d ed. Philadelphia, W. B. Saunders Co., 1993, p. 99.)

The *quantity* of x rays produced by the x-ray machine is controlled by the milliamperage and exposure time settings.

❐ Milliamperage settings are limited to 10 or 15 mA. More radiation is produced at higher mA settings.

❐ As exposure time increases, the amount of radiation to which the film and patient are exposed increases. Since both exposure time and milliamperage control the quantity of radiation that is generated, they may be expressed in combination as milliampere-seconds (mAs). To determine this value, multiply exposure time by the milliamperage setting.

---

mAs CALCULATION

- To determine milliampere-seconds (mAs), *multiply* the milliamperage setting by the exposure time.

  Formula: mA $\times$ exposure time = mAs

  Example: 15 mA at 2-second exposure time

  Solution: $15 \times 2 = 30$ mAs

  Example: 10 mA at 3-second exposure time

  Solution: $10 \times 3 = 30$ mAs

  Example: 15 mA at 120-impulse exposure time

  Solution: $15 \times {}^{120}\!/_{60} = 15 \times 2 = 30$ mAs

- To determine the exposure time required to achieve a given milliampere-second level, *divide* mAs by the mA.

  Formula: Exposure time = mAs/mA

  Example: 15 mA at __?__ seconds = 30 mAs

  Solution: ${}^{30}\!/_{15} = 2$ seconds exposure time

  Example: 10 mA at __?__ seconds = 30 mAs

  Solution: ${}^{30}\!/_{10} = 3$ seconds exposure time

- To determine the milliamperes required to achieve a given mAs, *divide* mAs by the exposure time:

Formula:	mA = mAs/exposure time
Example:	_?_ mA at 2 seconds = 30 mAs
Solution:	³⁰⁄₂ = 15 mAs
Example:	_?_ mA at 3 seconds = 30 mAs
Solution:	³⁰⁄₃ = 10 mAs

☐ It is preferable to use a higher milliamperage setting with a shorter exposure time. This reduces the chances of film or patient movement during the exposure.

☐ The amount of radiation reaching the film influences **film density,** which is the overall blackness of the film. It is measured by the amount of light which may be transmitted through the processed film. Density increases as the amount of radiation increases (Fig. 3-13).

The *quantity* of radiation reaching the film is also influenced by the distance between the target and the film. The terms used to describe the distance between the target and film are **tube–film distance (TFD),** *focal–film distance (FFD), target–surface distance (TSD),* and *target–film distance (TFD).* In this text, the term *tube–film distance (TFD)* will be used. TFDs commonly used in dental radiography are 8, 12, and 16 in. The 16-in TFD is preferred because it produces a sharper, less magnified image and less irradiated tissue. The TFD is determined by

☐ *The position of the tube in the tube head.* The tube may be positioned in the front or rear of the tube head. Rear positioning allows the use of a shorter, less cumbersome PID while retaining the desired TFD.

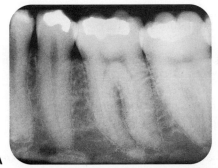 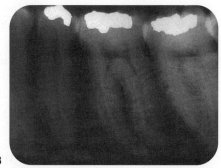

A   B

Figure 3-13. Density. Density is the overall blackness of the film. Note the increased density of film B.

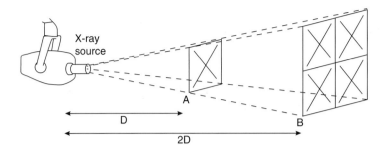

Figure 3-14. Intensity. As the distance from the target increases, the intensity of the x-ray beam (the number of x rays in a specific area) decreases. If the distance doubles, the intensity is one-quarter of the original intensity. If the distance is halved, the intensity is 4 times the original intensity.

❑ *The length of the PID.* The TFD increases as the length of the PID increases.

X rays produced at the target travel in straight lines which diverge increasingly as the distance from the target increases. As the distance from the target increases, the **intensity of the x-ray beam** (the number of x rays in a specific area) decreases (Fig. 3-14).

The *inverse-square law* states that the intensity of radiation is inversely proportional to the square of the distance from the source.

The quantity of radiation decreases in an area (such as at the film) as the distance from the target to the film increases. To produce an image with appropriate density, if changes are made in the length of the PID in use, changes also must be made in the amount of radiation produced. These changes are made in exposure time. The inverse-square law may be used to calculate exposure time.

INVERSE-SQUARE LAW CALCULATIONS

- The intensity of radiation is inversely proportional to the squares of the distances from the radiation source to the film.

   Formula: $\dfrac{\text{Intensity}_1}{\text{Intensity}_2} = \dfrac{(\text{distance}_2)^2}{(\text{distance}_1)^2}$

- Exposure time is proportional to the squares of the distances from the radiation source to the film.

   Formula: $\dfrac{\text{Exposure time}_1}{\text{Exposure time}_2} = \dfrac{(\text{tube–film distance}_1)^2}{(\text{tube–film distance}_2)^2}$

   Example: If the exposure time at a TFD of 8 in is 1 s, what will the exposure time (x) be at 16 in?

Solution:
$$\frac{1\ s}{x} = \frac{(8\ in)^2}{(16\ in)^2} = \frac{(1)^2}{(2)^2} = \frac{1}{4}$$
$$x = 4\ s$$

Example: If the exposure time at a TFD of 16 in is 20 impulses, what will the exposure time (x) be at 8 in?

Solution:
$$\frac{20\ impulses}{x} = \frac{(16\ in)^2}{(8\ in)^2} = \frac{(2)^2}{(1)^2} = \frac{4}{1}$$
$$20 = 4x$$
$$x = 5\ impulses$$

When changing TFD from 8 to 16 in, multiply the exposure time by 4.
When changing TFD from 16 to 8 in, divide the exposure time by 4.

III. INTRAORAL X-RAY FILM

Radiographic images are recorded on dental x-ray film.

A. Film Components

The film packet consists of the following components (Fig. 3-15):

❏ The *base* of dental x-ray film is clear plastic tinted blue to enhance image quality. It has an *embossed dot* in one corner to identify the side of the film that faced the radiation during exposure. The base provides strength and supports the emulsion.

❏ The *emulsion* is a coating on the base of the film which appears green when the film is unwrapped in daylight. Intraoral film is *double-emulsion film;* i.e., the film base is coated on both sides with emulsion. The emulsion contains *silver halide crystals,* which react to various types of energy, including radiation energy.

❏ The film is wrapped in *black paper* which assists in preventing light from reaching the film.

❏ Behind the film, on the side that faces away from the radiation source, is *lead foil,* which absorbs some primary radiation as well as backscattering secondary radiation that would fog the film.

❏ These components are all wrapped in a plastic material that prevents light and moisture from reaching the film. The side of the film packet which faces away from the radiation has a *colored tab* which is pulled to open the packet. The color of the tab is used to indicate the film speed and the number of films contained in the packet. Film packets

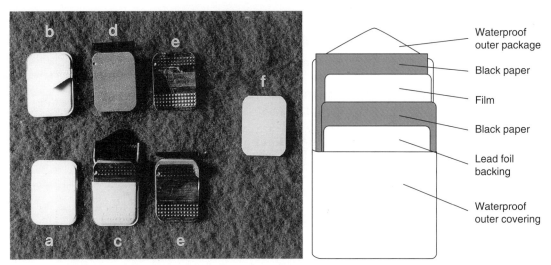

Figure 3-15. Film components. The outer plastic wrapper (a) prevents moisture and light from reaching the film. The back of the film (b) has a colored tab that opens the packet when pulled (c). The contents of the packet are wrapped in black paper (d). The lead foil (e) is located behind the film (f) in the packet.

may contain one or two films. Two-film packets are used when duplicate films are needed for patient records.

B. Film Speed

The size of the crystals in the emulsion affects the **film speed.** Larger crystals are more sensitive to radiation and require shorter exposure times. Crystal size also affects the sharpness of the radiographic image. Larger crystals produce less sharpness in the image. The slight decrease in sharpness in faster speed films (E speed) does not affect the diagnostic quality of the films. Crystal size is also referred to as *grain size.*

Since the exposure time required for E speed film is one-half that required for D speed film, it is recommended that E speed film be used for all intraoral exposures.

C. Film Size

Dental intraoral film packets are manufactured in sizes 0 to 4 (Fig. 3-16).

☐ *Size 0* (⅞ × 1⅜ in) is used for bitewing and periapical radiographs (see Chap. 4) on small children and also may be used for anterior periapical views on adults.

☐ *Size 1* (¹⁵⁄₁₆ × 1⁹⁄₁₆ in) may be used for periapical and bitewing radiographs on children 6 to 8 years old and for anterior periapical views on adults.

☐ *Size 2* (1¼ × 1⅝ in) is used for periapical radiographs on adults and children 9 years of age and older.

☐ *Size 3* (1⁹⁄₁₆ × 2⅛ in) is designed for bitewing examinations on adults

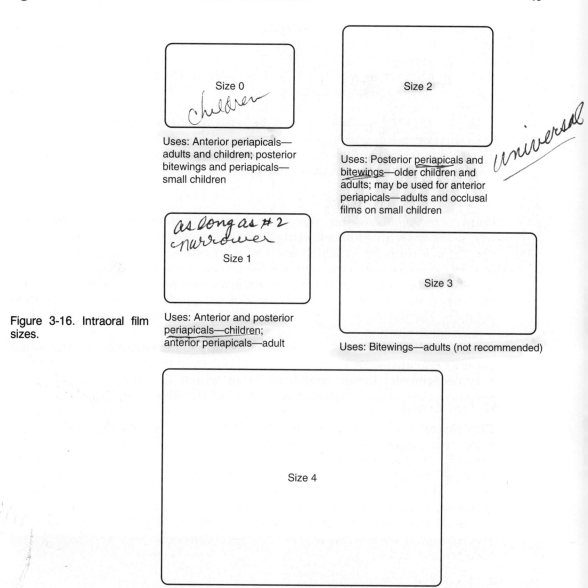

Size 0

children

Uses: Anterior periapicals—adults and children; posterior bitewings and periapicals—small children

Size 2

Uses: Posterior periapicals and bitewings—older children and adults; may be used for anterior periapicals—adults and occlusal films on small children

universal

as long as #2 narrower

Size 1

Figure 3-16. Intraoral film sizes.

Uses: Anterior and posterior periapicals—children; anterior periapicals—adult

Size 3

Uses: Bitewings—adults (not recommended)

Size 4

Occlusal films

and children 9 years of age and older. Its purpose is to eliminate the need for separate premolar and molar bitewing views. Its use is not recommended, as will be discussed in a later chapter.

☐ *Size 4* (2¼ × 3 in) is used for occlusal radiographs (see Chap. 11) on adults and children.

IV. FILM HOLDERS AND AIMING DEVICES

In order for the radiographic image to accurately represent the size, shape, and position of the teeth and other anatomic structures, the film must be positioned properly and the radiation beam must be aligned accurately with the teeth and film. The two intraoral techniques for film positioning and radiation beam alignment are the parallel technique and the bisecting the angle technique, which will be discussed in Chapters 8 and 9. Regardless of which technique is used, film holders or a combination of film holder and aiming device must be used. If a rectangular PID is used, film holders with aiming devices must be used to ensure proper alignment of the radiation beam and film.

There are many film holders and aiming devices available to practitioners. The following are those used most commonly.

A. The Stabe Film Holder

Constructed of disposable styrofoam, the *Stabe film holder* consists of a bite block with an attached upright that supports the film. In front of the upright is a thin slot in which the film is inserted. There is a groove on the bite block where it can be snapped off and shortened (Fig. 3-17).

The Stabe can be used for both anterior and posterior views. For anterior views, the film is inserted in the slot with its longest side in a vertical position. For posterior views, the film is positioned with its longest side in a horizontal position.

While the Stabe can be used for multiple radiographs on the same patient, it is advisable to prepare extra holders in the setup. The styrofoam may occasionally break, and the slot in which the film is inserted may become enlarged with repeated use, causing the film to slip.

❐ *Advantages*
  - Disposable
  - Inexpensive
  - Easy to use

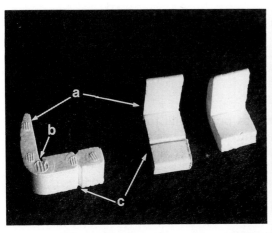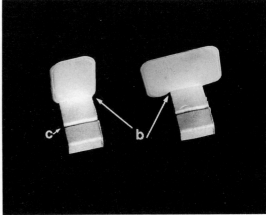

Figure 3-17. Stabe film holder. (a) The Stabe film holder consists of a bite block with an attached upright that supports the film. (b) In front of the upright is a thin slot in which the film is inserted. (c) There is a groove on the bite block where it can be snapped off and shortened. (Courtesy of Rinn Corporation, Elgin, Illinois.)

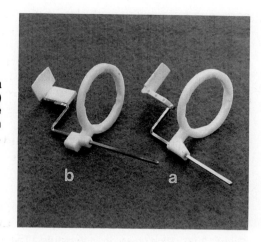

Figure 3-18. Rinn XCP. The Rinn XCP is a film holder and aiming device for anterior (a) and posterior (b) periapicals exposed with the parallel technique. When used with snap-on collimators, it provides rectangular collimation. (Courtesy of Rinn Corporation, Elgin, Illinois.)

- Easily tolerated by the patient
- Can be used with both the parallel and bisecting angle techniques

❑ *Disadvantages*
  - No aiming device
  - Cannot be used with rectangular collimation

B. The Rinn XCP Instrument

Designed for the parallel technique, The *Rinn XCP instrument* has a bite block of similar design to the Stabe. It is available in either styrofoam or autoclavable plastic (Fig. 3-18). A metal indicating arm attaches to the bite block and holds the aiming ring in position (Fig. 3-19). When used properly, the Rinn XCP instrument correctly aligns the film, teeth, and radiation beam for the parallel technique. Care must be taken to assemble the instrument properly and to position the film correctly in the patient's mouth.

The Rinn instrument may be used with round or rectangular PIDs. Round PIDs are aligned with the circular aiming ring. The corners of rectangular PIDs are aligned with notches on the circular aiming ring.

Rectangular collimating devices are available for Rinn instruments (Fig. 3-20). These flat, round metal disks with rectangular openings in the center snap on to the aiming ring to provide rectangular collimation for round PIDs.

Figure 3-19. Assembling the Rinn instrument. (Courtesy of Rinn Corporation, Elgin, Illinois.)

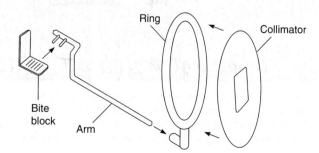

Bite block

Arm

Ring

Collimator

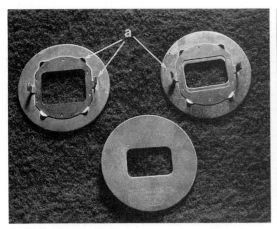 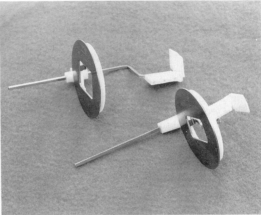

Figure 3-20. Rinn snap-on collimators. The Rinn snap-on collimators provide rectangular collimation when used with the XCP or BAI instruments. Clips on their back attach to the aiming ring (a). (Courtesy of Rinn Corporation, Elgin, Illinois.)

❏ *Advantages*
- Autoclavable or disposable
- May be used with rectangular collimation
- Component parts may be purchased separately
- Relatively inexpensive
- Easy to use
- Adjustable aiming ring
- Reduces technical errors

❏ *Disadvantages*
- May be assembled incorrectly
- Snap-on rectangular collimators are heavy, cannot be repositioned easily, and require extreme care in radiation beam alignment
- Care must be taken in film placement, since film placement errors result in beam alignment errors

C. The Rinn BAI Instrument

Designed for use with the bisecting angle technique, the *Rinn BAI instrument* is a film holder and aiming device (Fig. 3-21, left). Its autoclavable plastic bite block is similar to that of the XCP instrument except that it positions the film at an angle to the tooth instead of parallel to it and the area on which the patient bites is thicker (Fig. 3-21, right). When properly assembled and positioned, the BAI instrument correctly aligns the tooth, film, and radiation beam for the bisecting angle technique.

The bite blocks may be used with the XCP indicating arms and aiming rings. This allows the operator to easily switch to the bisecting angle technique in areas where the patient cannot accommodate parallel placement of the film, while using the preferred parallel technique for other

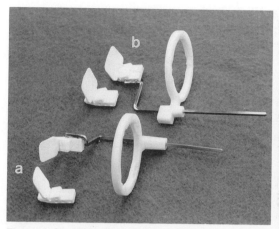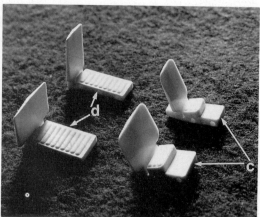

Figure 3-21. Rinn BAI. The Rinn BAI instrument is a film holder and aiming device for anterior (a) and posterior (b) periapicals exposed with the bisecting angle technique. When used with snap-on collimators, it provides rectangular collimation. The BAI's autoclavable plastic bite block (c) is similar to that of the XCP instrument (d) except that it positions the film at an angle to the tooth instead of parallel to it, and the area on which the patient bites is thicker. (Courtesy of Rinn Corporation, Elgin, Illinois.)

views. The bite blocks may be purchased separately, eliminating the need to purchase the entire BAI kit.

The BAI instrument may be used with round or rectangular PIDs or with the snap-on rectangular collimators, as may the XCP. The advantages and disadvantages are the same as those for the XCP instrument.

D. The Precision Instrument

The *Precision instrument* is a one-piece stainless steel film holder–aiming device–rectangular collimator combination (Fig. 3-22). As with the Rinn XCP instrument, it correctly aligns the film, teeth, and x-ray beam for the parallel technique when positioned properly. The only assembly required is addition of disposable plastic bite blocks, which increase patient comfort and aid the patient in securely gripping the instrument. Because of the

Figure 3-22. Precision instrument. The Precision instrument is a film holder and aiming device for anterior and posterior periapicals exposed with the parallel technique. The attached rectangular collimator provides rectangular collimation. (Courtesy of Masel Orthodontics, Bristol, Pennsylvania.)

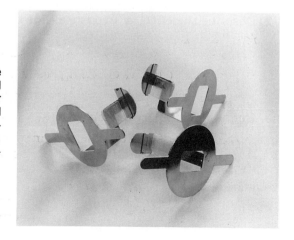

weight of the Precision instrument, the aiming ring–collimator has an extension that may be held to help support it while in place. The Precision instrument is completely autoclavable.

☐ *Advantages*
- Autoclavable
- No assembly required
- Provides rectangular collimation
- Reduces technical errors

☐ *Disadvantages*
- Expensive
- Heavy
- Patients may experience discomfort
- Cannot be used for bisecting the angle technique
- Plastic bite blocks may slip
- Aiming rings are not adjustable
- Require more careful radiation beam direction than rectangular
- Collimation achieved with rectangular PIDs

60 imp/sec

REVIEW EXERCISES

1. Make the following conversions in exposure time settings:

    ⅒ second = _6_ impulses

    ½ second = _30_ impulses

    12 impulses = _1/5_ seconds

    30 impulses = _1/2_ seconds

2. Describe the effect of exposure time on radiation production.

    Longer time = greater production of XR ie more impulses

3. Define milliampere-seconds (mAs).

    amperage is amount

4. Calculate milliampere-seconds for the following:

10 mA at 2-s exposure = _20_ mAs

15 mA at 1-s exposure = _15_ mAs

10 mA at 30 impulses = _5_ mAs

   10 " " ½ s

5. Identify the exposure times required to achieve the following milliampere-seconds:

15 mA at _⅓_ s = 5 mAs

10 mA at _½_ s = 5 mAs

10 mA at _30_ impulses = 5 mAs

6. Label the parts of the following x-ray tube:

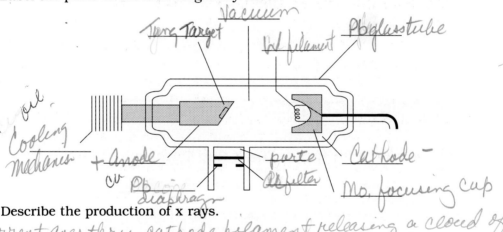

Tung Target   Vacuum   W filament   Pb glass tube

oil   Cooling mechanism   + Anode   Cu   Pb   diaphragm   Al filter   purte   Cathode −   Mo. focusing cup

7. Describe the production of x rays.

Current goes thru cathode filament releasing a cloud of electrons which are attracted to anode (+) hitting target & releasing energy in form of heat (99%) & x rays (1%)

8. Describe adjustments which influence x-ray quality and quantity.

Inc. Voltage creates higher energy XR, incr ma incr quantity of XR. Incr time also incr quantity ie quality ᵇ affecting quality.

9. State and explain the inverse-square law.

As the distance from the source of radiation increases the amount of radiation decreases proportionately ie to the sq of the dist

$$\frac{I_1}{I_2} = \frac{(D_2)^2}{(D_1)^2}$$

$$\frac{ET_1}{ET_2} = \frac{(TFD_1)^2}{(TFD_2)^2}$$

10. Use the inverse-square law to calculate the following exposure times:

   The exposure time at 8 in is ½ s. The exposure time at 16 in should be

   _2S_ . $\frac{1/2S}{X} = \frac{8^2}{16^2} = \frac{1/2}{X} = \frac{1^2}{2^2} = X = 2s$

   The exposure time at 16 in is 1 s. The exposure at 8 in should be _¼_ .

   $\frac{15 \cdot 1}{X} \cdot \frac{16^2}{8^2} = \frac{1}{X} = \frac{22}{12}$ $4X = 1$

   The exposure time at 8 in is 30 impulses. The exposure time at 16 in
   should be _2 S_ . $\frac{1/2S}{X} \quad \frac{8^2}{16^2} \quad \frac{1/2}{X} = \frac{1^2}{2^2} \quad X = 2$
   ___120 imp___

   The exposure time at 16 in is 60 impulses. The exposure at 8 in
   should be ___15 imp___. $\frac{16^2}{8^2} = \frac{1S}{X} \quad \frac{2^2}{1^2} = \frac{1}{X} \quad 4X = 1 \quad X = 1/4 S$

11. Define all the terms listed at the end of the Learning Objectives in this
    chapter.

LEARNING ACTIVITIES

Learning Activity 3-1: The X-Ray Machine

Equipment:

None

Location:

The x-ray operatory

Activity:

1. Identify the following, and describe the function of each:
   X-ray tube head _contains anode & cathode + wiring_
   Adjusting arm – _used for positioning_   _to produce XR_
   mA control – _adj quantity of XR_
   Voltmeter – _controls strength or "hardness" of X R_
   Timer – _length of exp_
   On/off switch –
   Position-indicating devices – _Rinn + Stabe_

Activating button — *make p*
Aluminum filter — *reduces soft XR & scatter*
Lead diaphragm — *reduces scatter & narrows beam.*
Number scale — *indicates amt of vert. angle ↑ – ↓+*

2. Demonstrate the following movements of the tube head:
   Adjust the vertical angulation to: +20, −20
   Make changes in horizontal angulation

3. Turn the x-ray machine on.

4. Demonstrate the following adjustments in kilovoltage:
   65, 70, 90.

5. Describe the effect of the preceding changes on the x-ray beam.

6. Change the mA setting from 10 to 15 mA.

Learning Activity 3-2: Intraoral X-Ray Film

Equipment:

5 dental x-ray films, sizes 0, 1, 2, 3, and 4

1 unexposed x-ray film (any size) processed in fix only (emulsion removed)

1 x-ray film (any size)

Activity:

1. Identify the five provided films by size, and describe the recommended use of each.

2. Unwrap a dental x-ray film (any size). Identify and describe the purpose of
   Color-coded opening tab — *indicate side away from XR & film speed.*
   Plastic wrap *protects & keeps dry*
   Black paper — *protects from light*
   Lead foil — *" " XR – some prim & secondary or scatter which is lead foil.*

3. Compare the unwrapped film with the provided film that has no emulsion.
   Describe the film emulsion and its effect on film speed and sharpness. *Is crystalline – lgr = faster & grainier*
   Describe the film base and its function. — *provides strength & supports emulsion. Blue tint enhances image quality*

Learning Activity 3-3: Film Holders/Aiming Devices

Equipment:

Rinn XCP and BAI instruments
Stabe film holders
Precision instrument/bite blocks

Activity:

1. Identify and assemble the following film holders/aiming devices:

   Rinn XCP

   Rinn BAI

   Stabe

   Precision instrument

2. Correctly place films in the preceding aiming devices for both anterior and posterior views.

3. Identify the area of the mouth in which Rinn and Precision instruments would be used.

4. Describe the advantages and disadvantages of the following film holders/aiming devices:

   Rinn XCP

   Rinn BAI

   Stabe

   Precision instrument

BIBLIOGRAPHY

Frommer, H. H. *Radiology for Dental Auxiliaries,* 5th ed. St. Louis, Mosby–Year Book, 1992.

Goaz, P. W., and White, S. C. *Oral Radiology Principles and Interpretation,* 2d ed. St. Louis, C.V. Mosby, 1987.

Miles, D. A., Van Dis, M. L., et al. *Radiographic Imaging for Dental Auxiliaries.* Philadelphia, W. B. Saunders Company, 1989.

Rinn Corp. *Intraoral Radiography with Rinn XCP/BAI Instruments.* Elgin, Ill., Rinn Corp., 1989.

The Full-Mouth Survey and Patient Management

4

After completing this chapter the student will be able to

1. Describe the rationale for taking a full-mouth series of radiographs on a patient.
2. Describe the types of film contained in a full-mouth survey.
3. Describe the appearance and purpose of periapical radiographs.
4. Describe the appearance and purpose of bitewing radiographs.
5. List the views contained in a full-mouth survey, the teeth that should appear in each, and the correct film size for each.
6. Describe the use of bitewing, periapical, occlusal, and panoramic films in pedodontic surveys.
7. Describe the rationale for exposing radiographs in edentulous areas.
8. Describe the use of occlusal, periapical, and panoramic films in edentulous surveys.
9. Describe factors that influence patient management, and list steps that will enhance the patient's experience.
10. Describe and demonstrate effective management of patients with a severe gag reflex.
11. Describe factors that influence children's behavior, and demonstrate effective management of the pedodontic patient.
12. Define the following terms:

Bitewing radiograph	Pedodontic
Clinical examination	Periapical radiograph
Edentulous	Radiograph
Full-mouth survey	

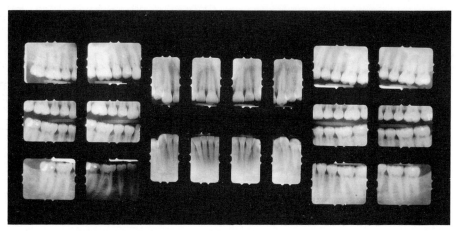

Figure 4-1. The adult full-mouth survey is composed of periapical and bitewing radiographs of all tooth-bearing areas in the mouth.

I. INTRAORAL SURVEYS

A. The Full-Mouth Survey

A dental **radiograph** is a special type of photographic image produced by the use of x rays and x-ray film. It allows the practitioner to see anatomic structures and pathology that would not otherwise be visible.

The **full-mouth survey** is a series of radiographs exposed in all teeth-bearing areas of the mouth *whether or not teeth are present* (Fig. 4-1). It demonstrates areas of the teeth, the surrounding bone, and underlying structures not visible in the clinical examination.

The **clinical examination** is a manual and visual assessment of the patient's head, neck, and oral cavity using examination instruments. It provides information about the condition of soft-tissue and tooth surfaces not visible in radiographs.

Both the clinical examination and the radiographic examination are necessary for a complete assessment and diagnosis of a patient's oral condition. Together they provide the practitioner with a total picture of the patient.

B. Component Radiographs

The full-mouth survey is composed of two types of radiographs:

❑ **Periapical radiographs** contain images of the entire tooth from the crown to 3 to 4 mm beyond the root apex (Fig. 4-2). Bone and anatomic structures surrounding the teeth are also visible. The full-mouth survey should include periapical radiographs of all tooth-bearing areas, since pathology may exist whether or not the teeth are present.

❑ **Bitewing radiographs** depict the crown and some of the root and surrounding bone of opposing *maxillary* and *mandibular* teeth on one film (Fig. 4-3). They are used primarily to examine the *proximal* surfaces of the teeth and to evaluate the *interproximal* bone. When all the

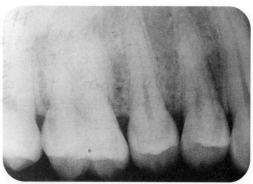

Figure 4-2. Periapical radiographs contain images of the entire tooth from the crown to 3 to 4 mm beyond the root apex.

teeth are present, premolar and molar bitewings are exposed. Vertical bitewings also may be included. Unlike periapical radiographs, it is only necessary to expose bitewings in areas where contacting and opposing teeth are present.

The need for radiographs is determined by the patient's age, dental history, and oral conditions. The ALARA concept must be followed. Exposure to ionizing radiation should always be considered and minimized; however, a complete and accurate diagnosis should never be jeopardized. The Department of Health and Human Services' guidelines (see Chap. 1, Table 1-4) should be followed in selecting the appropriate radiographic examination.

The number and size of the radiographs in a full-mouth survey will vary according to the dentist's training and personal preference. (Recommended uses for various film sizes are described in Chap. 3.) The adult full-mouth survey described in this text is a 20-film survey consisting of the following views exposed on both the right and left sides (Fig. 4-4):

☐ **Maxillary and mandibular anteriors.** Size 0 or 1 film may be used.

- *Central/lateral.* The central and lateral incisors are centered in the film. The mesial surfaces of the adjacent central incisor and canine should be visible.

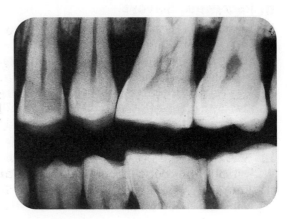

Figure 4-3. Bitewing radiographs depict the crown and some of the root and surrounding bone of opposing maxillary and mandibular teeth on one film.

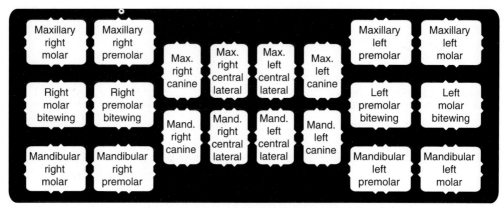

Figure 4-4. Radiographic views contained in the adult full-mouth survey.

- *Canine.* The canine is centered in the film. The distal aspect of the lateral incisor and the mesial aspect of the first premolar are visible.

☐ **Maxillary and mandibular posteriors.** Size 2 film is used.

- *Premolar.* Since the curvature of the arch prevents centering the premolars in the film, its anterior edge should be positioned at the middle of the canine. The distal aspect of the canine and the first molar should be seen as well as the premolars.

- *Molar.* The molar area is centered in the film. The anterior edge of the film is positioned at the middle of the second premolar. The distal aspect of the second premolar as well as the maxillary tuberosity or curvature of the ramus should be visible.

☐ **Bitewing radiographs.** Size 2 film is used.

- *Premolar.* The maxillary and mandibular premolar area from the distal aspect of the canines to the first molar should be visible.

- *Molar.* The maxillary and mandibular molar area from the distal aspect of the second premolars to the last molar should be visible.

C. Pedodontic Surveys

The **pedodontic** radiographic survey is a radiographic examination of the primary dentition, which contains only deciduous teeth, or the transitional dentition, which contains at least one permanent tooth in the presence of deciduous teeth.

Children are more sensitive to the effects of ionizing radiation than are adults. As with adult patients, routine radiographic surveys are not recommended. The Department of Health and Human Services' guidelines for patient selection should be followed. After a careful clinical examination, the type and number of radiographs required should be determined based on the patient's age, oral condition, and dental history.

The following types of films may be used alone or in combination as part of a pedodontic radiographic examination:

❏ *Bitewings* may be taken if the proximal surfaces of posterior teeth cannot be viewed clinically. Size 0, 1, or 2 film may be used depending on the age and size of the patient.

❏ *Periapicals* may be taken in selected areas of concern. Size 0, 1, or 2 film may be used depending on the age and size of the patient.

❏ *Occlusal films* may be exposed to view large areas of the maxilla or mandible in the assessment of dental disease, growth, and development. Large size 4 films are used to demonstrate an entire arch or a large area of an arch. Size 2 films may be used on small children.

❏ *Panoramic surveys* may be exposed to view the maxilla and mandible in the assessment of dental disease, growth, and development. They are large extraoral radiographs which demonstrate both the maxilla and mandible and surrounding anatomic structures on one film.

D. Edentulous Surveys

Retained roots, cysts, tumors, and other pathologic conditions may exist even when no teeth are present. For this reason, it is necessary to examine radiographically partially or completely **edentulous** areas (Fig. 4-5). The following radiographs may be used alone or in combination for this purpose:

❏ *Occlusal films* may be exposed to demonstrate large areas of an arch or an entire arch.

❏ *Panoramic surveys* may be taken to view both the maxilla and the mandible.

❏ *Periapical films* may be taken to view a specific area or may be taken in a series to view all teeth-bearing areas of the maxilla and mandible. Size 0, 1, or 2 film may be used for these purposes.

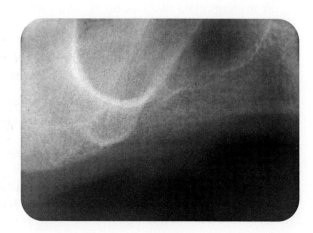

Figure 4-5. Radiographs must be exposed in all teeth-bearing areas of the mouth whether or not teeth are present.

II. PROFESSIONAL CONSIDERATIONS

A. Patient Management

The patient's perception of you as a professional plays a most important role in your ability to manage situations that may arise during an appointment. Regardless of your feelings, your demeanor must be calm, self-assured, organized, and professional at all times. The following techniques and appointment procedures will assist you:

❏ **Review the patient's record.** Personal, medical, and dental histories will provide information about fears, attitudes, and medical and dental conditions that may influence treatment and/or patient management procedures.

❏ **Be organized and prepared.** The operatory should be disinfected, wrapped, and ready for treatment when the patient arrives. Required equipment and films should be prepared and ready for use.

❏ **Establish rapport.** Talk with the patient. Introduce yourself, and briefly chat about nondental matters to help the patient relax.

❏ **Address the patient's concerns and questions.** Questions may arise about the procedure, sterilization and disinfection, or radiation hygiene. Listen carefully to the patient's concerns and questions. Address them factually using terminology the patient can understand.

❏ **Maintain a professional demeanor.** The anxiety that some patients experience in the dental setting may negatively influence their behavior. The behavior often can be managed with an assertive professional demeanor. However, a patient who is rude, uses profanity or abusive language, or is under the influence of alcohol or other drugs need not be tolerated. Advise the patient firmly and professionally that his or her behavior is unacceptable and that if it persists, he or she will be dismissed. In the case of intoxication or drug use, the patient should be dismissed but should be discouraged from driving. The assistance of your employer, co-worker, or a law enforcement officer may be required in managing or dismissing such a patient.

❏ **Do not tolerate sexual harassment.** Inappropriate remarks, touching, or other behavior that makes you uncomfortable should be handled firmly and professionally. The patient should be advised that his or her behavior is unacceptable and that if it persists, he or she will be dismissed. You may wish to seek assistance from your employer or a co-worker in managing or dismissing such a patient.

❏ **Place films carefully to minimize patient discomfort.** Work quickly and efficiently when exposing the radiographs
  • *Position the tube head and PID* in the approximate position before the film is placed. After film placement, only minor adjustments should be necessary.

- *Involve the patient.* If the x-ray machine makes a sound during the exposure, the patient may be advised to open his or her mouth and remove the film when the sound stops.

- *Begin exposures in the anterior region.* These are less likely to trigger the gag reflex.

- *Consider the patient's comfort while carefully placing the film.* Place the upper edge of the film in the deepest part of the palate for maxillary exposures. The upper corners of the film may be bent slightly for more comfortable placement.

- Mandibular exposures and bitewings should be placed away from the mandibular bone, especially in the premolar view. The floor of the mouth is more flexible as the film is moved lingually, allowing more comfortable film placement. This is especially true for patients with mandibular tori.

B. Controlling the Gag Reflex

Even the best preparation and procedures may fail in the presence of a severe gag reflex. Once triggered, it often cannot be stopped. Since it is a situation where "mind over matter" works, anything that you can do to assist the patient in focusing on something other than the procedure and gagging will help. Some strategies that may be helpful are

❑ Deep breathing through the nose.

❑ Focusing on a pleasant, calm place or a picture.

❑ Concentrating on keeping a leg or arm elevated during the exposure.

❑ Rinsing with anesthetic mouthwash or gargles.

The effectiveness of these strategies often depends on your ability to convince the patient of their effectiveness. If gagging persists, it may be necessary to reschedule the patient or, in extreme cases, take extraoral films.

C. Pedodontic Patient Management

The management of children during the x-ray appointment can either be a very rewarding or frustrating experience. As with adults, your demeanor can play a major role in achieving a successful outcome. Try to remember what it was like to be a child, what was fun and what was frightening (Fig. 4-6). Here are some tips for managing children:

❑ Children under age 4 may experience separation anxiety when the parent leaves. For this age group, it is best to have the parent present during treatment. In some instances, it may be necessary for the parent to hold the film in place.

❑ Older children usually will behave better if separated from the parent. Convincing the parent of this may offer a challenge in parent manage-

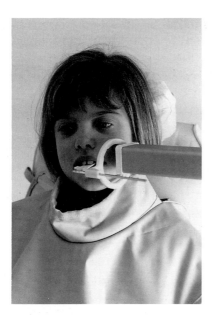

Figure 4-6. The management of children during the x-ray appointment can either be a very rewarding or frustrating experience.

ment! The child may be fearful of strangers, however. Take some time to get to know the child in the parent's presence. Then explain to the parent that it will be better for you to see the child alone and that he or she will be called if needed. Remember to be calm, firm, and professional.

☐ Children will be rested and more cooperative if their appointments are scheduled in the morning.

☐ Children are naturally curious and eager to learn about new things. However, they may be fearful of strange places and equipment. Explain things to them using language they can understand, but do not talk down to them or use "baby talk." The tube head and PID can be compared with a camera and the radiograph with a picture. Show children sample films and say that they may see their pictures when they are ready.

☐ Children love to play games, pretend, and be silly. Find the child inside you, and make a game of the appointment.

☐ Children find it very hard to sit still and are easily distracted. Remind them continuously of what they need to do.

☐ Children want to please and to do a good job. Use a lot of praise, and they will respond by working even harder for you.

☐ Children need clear limits for their behavior and will sense immediately if you are unsure of yourself. It is important to be in control of the appointment and to firmly, calmly, and professionally stop unacceptable behavior.

❑ Children who have had frightening medical experiences may associate clinical attire with those experiences and respond fearfully. Extra time may be needed with these patients for explanations and behavior management. Do not don masks, eyeglasses, and gloves until the explanations have been completed and treatment begins.

❑ With the exception of emergency situations when radiographs are needed immediately, it is better not to push the child if behavior problems persist. Try to understand the cause of the behavior (fear, fatigue, etc.), and address it calmly and firmly. Rescheduling at a time when the child is well rested may solve the problem. Remember that many fearful adult dental patients had bad dental experiences as children, and try to make the experience as nonthreatening and pleasant as possible.

REVIEW EXERCISES

1. Explain why a full-mouth survey is needed for patient assessment.

Demonstrates areas of teeth, bone & surrounding fundar tissue not visible on physical exa

2. Name and describe the types of films in an adult full-mouth survey. What is the purpose of each? *Cent & lat & canine PA, premolar & molar PA, premolar & molar bitewing. max & mand. ant, max & mand post, max & mand bitewing. size 0 or 1   size 2   size 2*

3. List the views that are contained in a full-mouth survey. What teeth should appear in each view? What size film is used for each?

Post. anterior peri apicals

View	Teeth	Film Size
R Ant Cent/lat incisor	mes edg 9, 8 7 mes edge 6 canine	0 or 1
LU " " " "	mes edge 8 9 10, mes edg canine	0 or 1
R low " " " "	27 26-25, 24	0-1
L M " " " "	25 24-23 22 Can.	0-1
R U Canine	Dist edg lat inc, Can, mes edg / premol.	0-1
R L Canine	" " " " " " " "	0-1
LU "	Dist edg lat inc, Can, mes edg / prem	0-1
LL "	" " " " " " "	0-1
RU pre mol.	mid edg Can - prem 1 & 2 - all of 1m	2
R L prem	mid edge " " " " " "	2
LU prem ol	" " " " " " " "	2
LL " "	" " " " " " " "	2
RU Molar	Dist edg of 2 pm - all mol - max tuberosity	2 2
RL "	or mand ramus	2 2
LU "		
LL "		

film upr / bih lat

*4 BWX - premolar - Dist edg can. - prem 1 & 2, mes edg 1m - 2 2
molar - Dist edg 2 prem - all molars - 2 2*

20 films

View	Teeth	Film Size

4. Describe how each of the following films may be used as part of a radiographic examination of a child.

   Bitewing

   Periapical

   Occlusal

   Panoramic

5. Describe the reasons for the edentulous radiographic survey.

6. Describe how each of the following films may be used in an edentulous radiographic survey.

   Occlusal

   Panoramic

   Periapical

7. Describe factors that influence patient management. List and describe the steps you can take to enhance the patient's experience.

8. Think about and then describe what you might do to manage the following patients.

   An intoxicated patient

   A hostile patient who uses profanity

   A patient who speaks suggestively to you about sexual matters

9. Describe techniques for managing the gag reflex.

10. Describe behavioral characteristics of the pedodontic patient. What methods would you use to manage a child exhibiting each of the characteristics?

11. Define all the terms listed at the end of the Learning Objectives in this chapter.

LEARNING ACTIVITIES

Learning Activity 4-1: Patient Management

Equipment:

None

Activity:

Describe what you might do in the following situations. Take some time to think about your response.

Situation 1:
After you seat your patient, she says, "I've heard that you can get AIDS in the dental office. What do you do to prevent this from happening?"

Your response:

Situation 2:
You are about to expose a full-mouth survey on your patient when he says, "I had a chest x ray last month. Should I be having x rays again this soon?"

Your response:

Situation 3:
You notice the odor of alcohol on your patient's breath, his eyes are bloodshot, and his speech is slurred. You are having difficulty exposing the films because the patient is unable to follow your directions and his movements are erratic.

Your response:

Situation 4:
Your patient is your employer's best friend and golfing partner. He is a prominent attorney in your town. As you reach across him to move the x-ray tube head, he touches you and whispers, "I'd like to see more of you. Meet me for a drink after work."

Your response:

Situation 5:
Your patient is a 7-year-old boy with a doting mother. They are new to the dental practice where you are employed. The boy's mother tells you that she always stays with him during his appointments.

Your response:

Situation 6:
Your patient is a 4-year-old girl who needs bitewing radiographs. This is her first dental visit.

Your response:

BIBLIOGRAPHY

Frommer, Herbert, H. *Radiology for Dental Auxiliaries,* 5th ed. St. Louis, Mosby–Year Book, 1992.

Goaz, P. W., and White, S. C. *Oral Radiology.* St. Louis, C.V. Mosby, 1987.

The Darkroom:
Processing the Radiograph

After completing this chapter the student will be able to

1. Describe latent image production.
2. Describe the effect of exposure time, mA, and kVp (kilovolts) on film density.
3. Describe the effect of film density and kVp on film contrast.
4. Describe darkroom design specifications, including

    Factors to consider in darkroom design

    Light-tight entrance designs

    Lighting requirements

    Safelighting requirements

    Construction materials

    Plumbing requirements
5. Identify and describe the correct use of processing equipment, including

    Manual film processing equipment

    Automatic film processing equipment

    Lighting/safelighting

    View box

    Timer

    Thermometer

    Film duplicator

    Stepwedge

    Film hangers

    Film dryer

    Film stirrers
6. Identify the chemical components of developer and fix solutions, and describe their action.

7. Describe factors that influence the life of processing solutions.

8. Describe and demonstrate solution preparation and replenishment procedures.

9. Identify state and local regulations for the disposal of processing chemicals and lead foil.

10. Describe and demonstrate the time-temperature method of film processing.

11. Describe and demonstrate automatic film processing.

12. Describe and demonstrate darkroom and equipment maintenance procedures.

13. Describe and demonstrate quality assurance procedures for

    Solution testing

    Safelight testing

    Light-leak testing

14. Describe and demonstrate proper film storage.

15. Define the following terms:

    Contrast   Scale of contrast

    Film Density   Wet reading

    Latent image

Films exposed using the most careful radiographic technique may be ruined with careless or faulty processing procedures. Darkroom design and cleanliness, film storage, solution temperature and quality, equipment functioning, and operator technique influence the quality of the finished radiograph. Careful attention must be paid to each of these factors to produce radiographs of optimal quality.

I. THE DARKROOM

A. Darkroom Design

The floors, counters, and cabinets of the darkroom should be constructed of easily cleaned, chemical- and water-resistant materials. The walls should be washable, resistant to chemicals and water, and painted a light color to reflect safelighting.

The following factors also should be considered in the design of a darkroom:

❏ **Traffic.** Determine the maximum number of people requiring use of the darkroom at a given time. Will it be in a large clinic, where several clinicians may be using it simultaneously, or will it be in a small office, where only one person will process films at a given time?

❏ **Processing requirements.** Determine the maximum number of films processed each day. Will manual and/or automatic processing be used? Will space be required for film drying and the duplication of films?

❑ **Storage requirements.** What kind of storage space is needed? Materials that produce dust or chemical fumes must not be stored in the darkroom, nor should open packages of film be stored in the darkroom to avoid possible contamination by the processing solutions.

Film should be stored at 50 to 70°F at 30 to 50 percent humidity. Its expiration date should be clearly visible, and the supply should be rotated so that older film is used first. Film also should be protected from radiation exposure.

[handwritten margin note: including refrig. and radiation shield from insulation]

❑ **Location.** The darkroom should be located near all x-ray units, providing convenient access for all.

❑ **Size.** The preceding considerations will assist in determining the size of the darkroom. It is important that the darkroom be large enough to accommodate present needs as well as any future growth of the facility. It should be no smaller than 4 × 4 ft.

❑ **Design.** The darkroom must be free from any *light leaks*—white light that enters the darkroom through openings around doors or other structures.

The darkroom also should be protected from accidental door openings during processing. X-ray film is sensitive to white light as well as radiation (see Radiographic Image Formation, below). Three types of entrances prevent light exposure during processing:

❑ A weatherstripped door equipped with a lock and/or an outside light to indicate that processing is in progress. There is no access to the darkroom during processing.

❑ A light-tight revolving cylinder with an opening on one side may be turned to allow freedom of movement in and out of the darkroom during processing.

❑ A maze design provides access to the darkroom through a turning corridor painted matte black to prevent the reflection of white light. It allows freedom of movement in and out of the darkroom during processing. However, more space is required to accommodate this design (Fig. 5-1).

B. Darkroom Lighting

Darkroom lighting should include

❑ **An overhead white light.** This is for illumination of the darkroom. It should be located where it will not be turned on accidentally during processing.

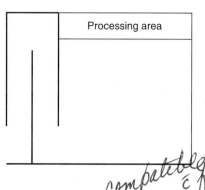

Figure 5-1. Maze-design darkroom. A maze design provides access to the darkroom through a turning corridor painted matte black to prevent the reflection of white light.

compatible c̄ film used.

☐ **A safelight.** This is a light equipped with a low-watt light bulb and a red or yellow filter to eliminate the blue-green part of the light spectrum to which x-ray film is sensitive. The filter must be adequate for the most sensitive films used in the facility (Fig. 5-2).

- A Kodak yellow Morlite M-2 filter equipped with a 7.5- to 10-W light bulb placed no closer than 3 ft from the work surface is appropriate for intraoral films but not for more sensitive extraoral screen film.

- A Kodak GBX-2 safelight filter with at 15-W bulb may be used with extraoral screen films and intraoral films. It should be positioned 3 to 4 ft from the work surface. *where you unwrap film.*

☐ **A radiograph view box.** This is convenient for **wet readings,** that is, for viewing films after they have been fixed for 3 minutes (see Fig. 5-2).

NO! because fluorescent tubes flicker on and off after turning off

☐ **An outside warning light.** Lit during processing, this helps to prevent accidental door opening during processing.

C. Darkroom Plumbing

Darkroom plumbing should include (see Fig. 5-2)

☐ A stainless steel sink equipped with a gooseneck faucet to allow cleaning of solution tanks and other equipment.

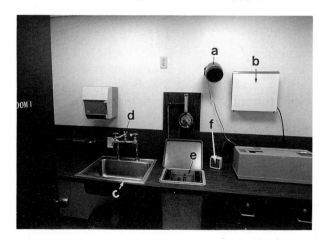

Figure 5-2. Darkroom setup. (a) Safelight. (b) View box. (c) Sink. (d) Faucet. (e) Tanks. (f) Timer.

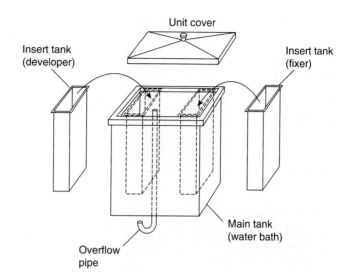

Figure 5-3. Typical manual processing tanks.

□ Hot and cold water lines that provide thermostatically controlled water for processing.

□ Chemical-resistant drain plumbing.

D. Equipment

A properly equipped darkroom facilitates processing and helps to eliminate errors. It should include the following:

□ **Processing tanks.** These are usually 1-gal stainless steel tanks suspended in a larger stainless steel tank containing circulating water at a constant temperature (68 to 70°F). The tank containing the developing solution is most commonly suspended on the left side of the larger tank, the fixer tank on the right. A water bath for film rinsing is between the two tanks. Water circulates around the tanks to maintain a constant solution temperature. A drain is located at the bottom of the large tank into which a tall drainpipe is inserted during processing to keep the water flowing at solution-top level (Fig. 5-3).

□ **Timer.** An accurate timer must be used to determine the correct processing time based on solution temperature (see Fig. 5-2).

□ **Thermometer.** An accurate thermometer should be suspended in the developing solution and checked prior to processing any films (Fig. 5-4). If the temperature of the developer is not at 68 to 70°F, the temperature of the water bath should be checked and adjusted. Time must be allowed for the temperatures to equalize, especially if the tanks have not been used for a period of hours. Processing should not occur until the correct temperature is reached.

□ **Film hangers.** Film hangers are used to hold films in the processing solutions (Fig. 5-5A). Various types are available, the most common

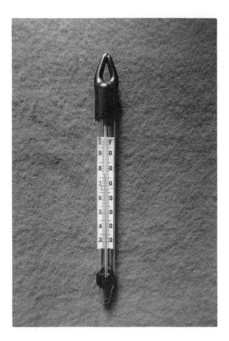

Figure 5-4. Thermometer. An accurate thermometer is essential for manual processing.

being a stainless steel hanger with 1 to 20 clips to which films are attached. The top of the hanger is curved so that it may be hung on the side of the processing tank. Hangers may be equipped with plastic tags for labeling.

☐ **Dryer/drying racks.** To dry the films after processing, the film hangers may be hung on bars placed in the darkroom for this purpose,

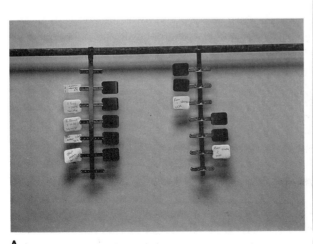

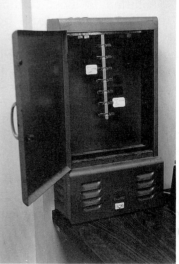

A   B

Figure 5-5. Film dryers and/or drying racks are necessary for manual processing. **(A)** Film hangers on drying racks. **(B)** Dryer.

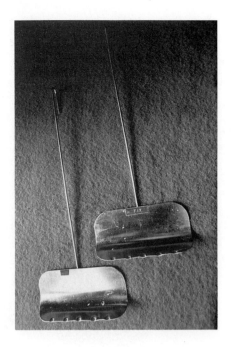

Figure 5-6. Stirrers. Solutions stirrers are required for stirring the solutions in manual processing.

or they may be hung in drying cabinets which circulate warm air around the films for faster drying (Fig. 5-5). Films should be hung away from the work area, where they may be contaminated by chemicals or dust.

☐ **Solution stirrers.** These come in various designs. They are used to stir the solutions prior to processing because the chemicals in the solution tend to concentrate at the bottom of the tank (Fig. 5-6).

II. RADIOGRAPHIC IMAGE FORMATION

The black and white radiographic image is created when radiation strikes the film, energizing silver halide crystals suspended in its emulsion (see Chap. 3). The crystals also may be energized by other forms of energy, such as heat, light, electricity, chemicals, and pressure.

A pattern of energized crystals called the **latent image** is created by the different amounts of radiation passing through structures of different densities. Dense objects such as teeth, bone, and metal restorations absorb radiation and prevent it from reaching the film, thereby energizing few crystals. Objects that absorb radiation are *radiopaque.* Low-density objects, such as lips, cheeks, and gingiva, allow radiation to pass through, thereby energizing many crystals. Objects that do not absorb radiation are *radiolucent.*

During the development process, the silver from the energized crystal is deposited in the emulsion as black metallic silver. This creates black and dark gray radiolucent areas. Crystals that have not been energized are removed from the emulsion during the fixing process, creating clear and light gray radiopaque areas (Fig. 5-7).

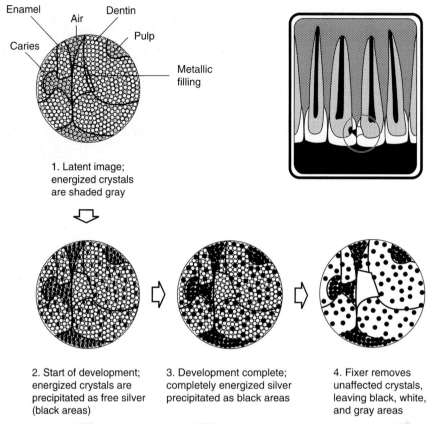

1. Latent image;
energized crystals
are shaded gray

2. Start of development;
energized crystals are
precipitated as free silver
(black areas)

3. Development complete;
completely energized silver
precipitated as black areas

4. Fixer removes
unaffected crystals,
leaving black, white,
and gray areas

Figure 5-7. Latent image production and the action of processing chemicals.

III. RADIOGRAPHIC FILM QUALITIES: DENSITY AND CONTRAST

A. Density

The degree of overall blackness in the processed film is called **density** (Fig. 5-8). It is measured by the amount of light that may be transmitted through the film. The density of the processed radiograph is influenced by

☐ **The quantity of radiation reaching the film.** If more radiation reaches the film, more crystals will be energized and deposited in the emulsion during processing.

* *Milliamperage (mA) and exposure time* are the primary factors influencing film density. Both affect the amount of radiation emitted from the x-ray machine and therefore influence image density.

* *Kilovoltage (kVp)* affects the penetrating power of the x-ray beam. If the beam is not powerful enough to penetrate tissues, it will not reach the film and energize the silver halide crystals. Kilovoltage can affect film density by influencing the amount of radiation reaching the film.

* *The thickness and density of the object* influence the amount of radiation absorbed and therefore the amount of radiation reaching

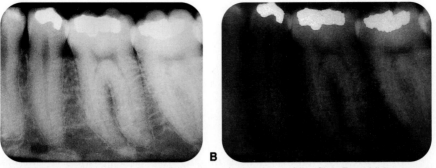

Figure 5-8. Film density. Film **A** exhibits normal density, while film **B** exhibits excessive density.

(at. mass)

the film. The thicker and the denser the object, the more radiation is absorbed.

❏ **Processing time.** Processing for too short a time will result in a light film because all the energized crystals will not have time to precipitate into the emulsion. Processing for too long a time may cause excessive silver precipitation, resulting in a film that is too dark.

❏ **Processing temperature.** Temperature affects the activity of the developing agents and the amount of time required to complete processing. At high temperatures, shorter developing times are needed because the developing agents are very active. If the processing time is not altered at high temperatures, the films will be overdeveloped and too dark. At low temperatures, the developing agents work slowly or may be inactive. Failure to lengthen the developing time at low temperatures results in a light, underdeveloped film.

B. Contrast

The ability of the film to demonstrate varying degrees of radiation absorption by structures of different densities is called **contrast.** It appears in the radiograph as gradations in shades of gray from black to white.

❏ A short **scale of contrast** (high contrast) occurs when the film exhibits very black areas and white areas with few shades of gray (Fig. 5-9).

❏ A long scale of contrast (low contrast) occurs when the film exhibits many shades of gray as well as black and white (Fig. 5-9).

Contrast in the radiograph is influenced by

❏ **Film density.** If the film is too dark or too light, contrast in the film will not be visible.

❏ **Radiation quality.** The quality of the radiation produced by the x-ray machine affects its ability to penetrate objects. Radiation must have

KvP / CONTRAST

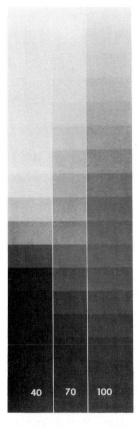

Figure 5-9. Scale of contrast appears in the radiograph as gradations in shades of gray from black to white. A short scale of contrast (high contrast) occurs when the film exhibits very black areas and white areas with few shades of gray *(left band)*. A long scale of contrast (low contrast) occurs when the film exhibits many shades of gray as well as black and white *(right band)*. The scale of contrast in a radiograph increases as the kilovoltage increases. (From Miles DA, et al: *Radiographic Imaging for Dental Auxiliaries,* 2d ed. Philadelphia. W.B. Saunders Company, 1993. P. 99.)

sufficient penetrating power to pass through structures of varying densities and thicknesses so that the film may demonstrate the different amounts of radiation that they absorb. Kilovoltage controls the quality of the radiation and the amount of contrast in the radiograph. At a higher kVp setting, the radiation produced has more penetrating power than that produced at a low kVp setting. Because filtration removes less powerful x rays from the radiation beam and leaves the more powerful x rays, adding filtration also increases the scale of contrast in the radiograph.

IV. PROCESSING THE RADIOGRAPH

Radiographic processing is a chemical reaction that transforms the latent image into a visible image. It may be done manually, using the time-temperature method, or automatically, using an automatic film processing unit. Regardless of the processing method, similar processing chemicals are used. For an optimal chemical reaction, it must occur during a specific time interval at a specific temperature.

A. Processing Solutions

There are two solutions needed to process a radiograph (Table 5-1):

❐ The *developing solution* contains chemicals that cause the silver in the energized crystals to precipitate out of the crystal while the halides

Table 5-1. Processing Solutions

alkaline or basic (handwritten)

Chemical	Function	Action
Developer: Chemicals and Their Action *reducing agent = alkaline or basic* (handwritten)		
Elon or Metol	Developing agents	Bring out image quickly, produces low contrast, not temperature sensitive
Hydroquinone	Developing agent	Builds up contrast slowly during development, very active at high temperatures
Sodium sulfite	Preservative	Prevents oxidation
Sodium carbonate	Activator	Provides alkaline medium, softens gelatin to allow developing agents to reach silver bromide crystals
Potassium bromide	Restrainor	Controls activity of developing agents, prevents chemical fog
Fixer: Chemicals and Their Action		
Sodium thiosulfate (hyposulfate)	Fixing agent	Removes unexposed or undeveloped silver bromide crystals from emulsion
Sodium sulfite	Preservative	Prevents deterioration of hypo and precipitation of silver
Potassium alum (potassium aluminum sulfate)	Hardening agent	Shrinks and hardens gelatin
Acetic acid	Acidifier	Provides acid medium

rinse about 20 sec. in manual proc. (handwritten)

acetic (handwritten)

are released as gas. The precipitated silver creates the dark (radiolucent) areas of the radiographic image. Crystals that have not been energized are not affected by the developing solution. The following chemicals are contained in the developing solution:

- The developing agents, energized *elon* and *hydroquinone,* cause the precipitation of silver from the silver halide crystal. Hydroquinone brings out the contrast in the image. It is inactive under 60°F and very active over 70°F. Processing at low temperatures produces low contrast in the radiographic image, and processing at high temperatures results in high contrast. Elon, which is not as temperature sensitive, quickly brings out the shades of gray in the image.

- The preservative, *sodium sulfite,* extends the life of the developing agents by deterring their oxidation.

- The activator, *sodium carbonate,* provides the necessary alkaline medium required for the chemical action of the developing agents. It also softens and swells the emulsion, allowing the developing agents to reach the energized crystals.

- The restrainer, *potassium bromide,* slows down the action of the developing agents and deters their action on unexposed crystals, thereby preventing chemical fog.

❑ The *fixing solution* contains *=clearing agent* (handwritten) chemicals that remove the undeveloped silver halide crystals and harden the emulsion.

- The fixing agent (also known as the clearing agent), *sodium thiosulfate,* is also called *hypo.* It removes all silver halide crystals from the emulsion. — *giving the radiopaque area.* (handwritten)

- The acidifier, *acetic acid,* creates an acid medium to neutralize and inhibit any developing solution carried to the fixing solution.

- The preservative, *sodium sulfite,* is the same chemical preservative found in the developer. It extends the life of the fixing solution by inhibiting deterioration of the fixing agent and preventing oxidation of any developer that may remain on the film.

- The hardening agent, *potassium alum,* shrinks and hardens the emulsion.

B. Solution Preparation, Maintenance, and Disposal

☐ **Solution preparation.** Processing solutions are available commercially for both manual and automatic processing. The manual processing solutions are usually concentrated, producing 1 gal of solution when diluted with water. Automatic solutions are available prepared or in concentrate form. Manufacturers directions should be followed in the preparation of all solutions.

☐ **Solution maintenance.** Small amounts of processing solution are lost during processing and through evaporation. Oxidation takes place as the solutions are exposed to air, and the solution becomes "exhausted." Exhaustion of the developer is demonstrated by a light, "thin" image; the density of the radiograph is decreased when compared with films processed in newly prepared solution. Exhaustion in the fixer solution is demonstrated by an increase in the amount of time that is required for the film to clear. Factors that influence the life of processing solutions are as follows:

- *Care in initial preparation.* The solutions must be carefully prepared and poured into containers that have been scrupulously cleaned and rinsed. Tanks and containers should be cleaned with a mild detergent and soft brush whenever solutions are changed. To avoid solution contamination, separate brushes and cleaning devices must be identified and used for each solution. Care must be taken to always use the same container for each solution.

- *Maintenance/replenishment (automatic processors).* The maintenance and replenishment of automatic processing solutions vary with different models and manufacturers. Always carefully follow the manufacturer's directions for cleaning and replenishing.

- *Maintenance/replenishment (manual processing). Cover* manual processing tanks whenever they are not in use to reduce evaporation and oxidation. Care should be taken to always place the tank cover in the same position over the tanks. This will avoid contamination of the solutions caused by the condensation of developer or fixer on the cover dripping into the wrong solution. *Replenish* solutions daily by removing 8 oz of each solution and adding fresh solution to the fill line on the side of the tank. Commercially prepared replenishers are available, or gallon containers of the standard processing solutions may be prepared when the solutions are changed and used for replenishing until the next scheduled solution change.

- *Volume of films processed.* Each time a film is processed, the solutions are weakened. Therefore, the number of films processed daily affects the life of the solutions. Most facilities will require a change in solutions every 2 to 4 weeks. A schedule for solution change should be established and posted for each facility. Each solution change should be noted and signed by the person responsible. Solution testing should occur daily after replenishment (see Quality Control: Solution Testing). Regardless of the established schedule, solutions should be changed if this test so indicates.

☐ **Quality control: solution testing.** The quality of the processing solutions should be tested daily after they have been replenished.

- *Stepwedge/Stepwedge construction.* To test the solutions, a stepwedge is needed. It may be purchased or constructed from layers of lead foil from film packets. A purchased stepwedge is constructed of increasing thicknesses of aluminum, giving it the appearance of a tiny aluminum staircase (Fig. 5-10). A simple stepwedge may be constructed by taping increasing layers of lead foil from film packets to a piece of firm cardboard or a tongue depressor: The first step is one layer of foil; the second step, two layers; and the third step, five layers of foil. When a stepwedge is placed on a film and the film is exposed and processed, the density of the steps will decrease as the step thicknesses increase. This is due to the increased amounts of radiation absorbed by the increased thicknesses of the steps.

- *Preparation of test films.* Prepare sufficient films for processing one each day until the next scheduled solution change. Expose each film by placing it on a surface convenient to the x-ray machine with the stepwedge on top of it. Place the PID 1 to 2 in away,

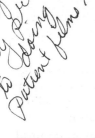

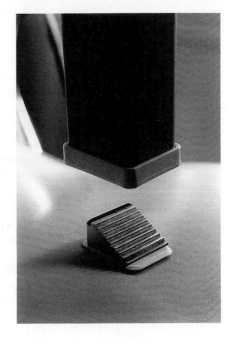

Figure 5-10. Stepwedge exposure technique. Place the stepwedge on the film with the PID 1 to 2 in away so that additional exposures may be made without moving the PID. Expose each film at the same exposure settings.

allowing enough space to ensure that after each film is exposed, it may be removed and the next put in its place without altering the position of the PID (see Fig 5-10). Expose each film at the same exposure settings. By exposing the films at the same settings and tube-film distance, exposure variables are eliminated. Any changes in the appearance in the films will be due to processing variables.

- *Processing the films.* Process the control film after changing the solutions. Label it and tape it to the darkroom viewbox or place it on a hanger for comparison with the remaining films. Refrigerate the remaining films to avoid film changes due to alterations in temperature. Process one each day after replenishing, stirring, and adjusting the temperature of the solutions. Compare each film with the control film. If a visible decrease in the density of the steps occurs (a two-step decrease if an aluminum stepwedge is used), the solutions must be changed.

❏ **Solution disposal/silver retrieval and scrap foil disposal.** State and federal regulations must be followed in the disposal of processing chemicals. The residual silver contained in the fixing solution may prohibit its dumping into the sewer system. Silver retrieval systems are available which remove silver by chemical precipitation or electrolysis. Companies that specialize in the collection and disposal of hazardous waste will provide containers and a routine pickup schedule. The local environmental protection agency and public health department can provide guidelines for your area. Lead foil from film packets should be saved and recycled. The same companies that pick up processing chemicals or scrap amalgam may provide disposal services for the foil.

C. Manual Processing with the Time-Temperature Method

The time-temperature method of film processing is used for manual film processing. Films are developed for a specific amount of time based on the temperature of the developer.

1. The films are placed in the developer.
   Note: The time-temperature combinations at which the developer produces the best radiographic image are developing for 4 minutes at 70°F or developing for 4½ minutes at 68°F. However, acceptable radiographs can be produced at higher temperatures if the developing time is decreased and at lower temperatures if the developing time is increased (Table 5-2). Since the ideal temperatures for processing are 68 to 70°F, every effort should be made to process within this temperature range.

2. After developing the radiographs, the films are rinsed by moving the hanger up and down in the water bath 10 to 20 times. This removes the developer from the film and stops further development.

3. The films are next placed in the fixer solution for 10 minutes. They will have cleared (lost their cloudy appearance) after approximately 3 minutes in the fixer.

temp up — time down & conversely

Table 5-2. Developer Time-Temperature Combinations

	Developer Temperature	Film Immersion Time
Lower temperatures	60°F	6 min
	65°F	5 min
Optimal temperature range	68°F	4½ min
	70°F	4 min
Higher temperatures	75°F	3 min
	80°F	2½ min

Note: Since the crystals can be energized by white light prior to clearing, always check for clearing under safelight conditions. After the films have cleared, they may be read, if necessary. This wet reading must be followed by fixing for the remaining amount of time or the quality of the image will deteriorate over time.

→ circulating water

4. After fixing, the films are placed in the water bath for 20 minutes to remove any remaining fixer solution.
   Note: If the films are not thoroughly washed, residual fix will stain the films brown over a period of time, reducing the quality of the image.

5. The films are next dried in dryer or at room temperature. They must be thoroughly dry before handling.
   Note: Throughout processing, care must be taken in film handling:
   • Follow infection-control guidelines (see Chap. 2).
   • Handle film as little as possible with clean, dry hands; touch only outer edges.
   • Do not let films touch in processing tanks. This will prevent the solution from reaching the areas of the film that are in contact. Scratching of the emulsion may occur if the films rub against other films during processing.
   • Avoid film contact with dust or chemicals by maintaining a clean darkroom.

D. Automatic Processing

There are many different models of automatic processors on the market (Fig. 5-11). Simple models have containers of processing solutions and water that require regular maintenance and replenishing. Plumbing is required for more complex models which have a constant water flow. Some models automatically replenish the solutions each time a film is processed. Before using an automatic processor, carefully read the manufacturer's directions.

❑ **Automatic processor design.** While the models may differ, the basic design of automatic processors is the same (Fig. 5-12):
   • The *transport system,* usually rollers, moves the film along through the chemicals and water bath. Special squeegee rollers remove excess chemicals, reduce carry-over from one solution to the next, and remove excess water prior to drying.

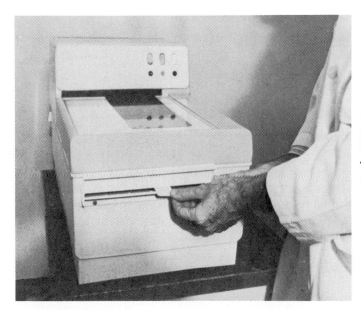

Figure 5-11. Automatic processor. (From Frommer HH: *Radiology for Dental Auxiliaries,* 5th ed. St. Louis, Mosby–Year Book, 1992. P. 103.)

- The *heater* maintains a constant temperature in the developer. Temperatures in automatic processing range from 74 to 105°F depending on the model used. *most 80-85°*

- The *dryer* circulates warmed air around the film to speed drying.

- The *daylight loader* attaches to the automatic processor and permits film loading in white light conditions. The top of the daylight loader is a filter similar to the safelight filter. Hands are inserted into the loader through light-tight sleeves. Film unwrapping and loading can be observed through the filter. The risk of cross-contamination is high with the use of daylight loaders. They should only be used with film wrappers that are removed before the films are placed in the daylight loader. Careful handwashing and infection-control procedures must be followed.

❑ **Maintenance.** To avoid equipment breakdown and damaged films, careful maintenance of the automatic processor is essential. A cleaning and replenishment (if needed) schedule should be established based on

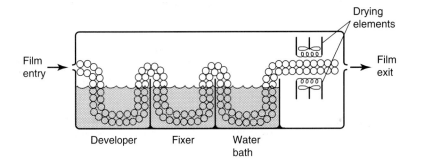

Figure 5-12. Automatic processor design.

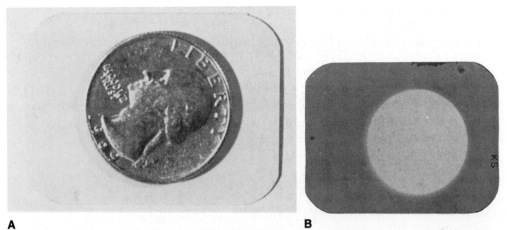

A　　　　　　　　　　　　　　　　　　　**B**

Figure 5-13. Coin test for safelighting. **(A)** Coin placed on unexposed film under safelight. **(B)** Developed film showing outline of coin, indicating that safelight intensity is too great and not safe. (From Frommer HH: *Radiology for Dental Auxiliaries,* 5th ed. St. Louis, Mosby–Year Book, 1992. P. 89.)

the number of films processed daily. Follow the manufacturer's directions for these procedures.

❐ **Processing.** Automatic processing reduces the time required for a finished radiograph from approximately 1 hour to 4 to 5 minutes. It simplifies the processing procedure as well. Carefully unwrap the films following infection-control procedures (see Chap. 2). Slowly feed the films into the processor, counting 10 to 15 seconds between each.

E. Testing for Light Leaks

White light leaking into the darkroom during processing will result in film fog in the radiographic image. To check for light leaks, stand in the darkroom with all doors closed and lights off until your eyes adjust to the dark. Look around the room for slivers of white light. They usually occur around doors, electrical fixtures, or wall joints. All light leaks must be sealed with weather stripping or caulking.

F. Safelight Testing

To test for proper safelight conditions, perform the *coin test.* With no light, unwrap an unexposed film and place it on the darkroom counter where films are usually unwrapped and placed on hangers. Place a penny or other coin on the film, and turn on the safelight. Leave the coin in place for 5 to 7 minutes, and then process the film. If the outline of the coin appears, the crystals in the area uncovered by the coin have been energized (Fig. 5-13). This may be due to an incorrect or damaged safelight filter, a safelight placed too close to the work surface, or a safelight bulb that is too strong for the filter. Safelighting should be tested periodically because the filters may deteriorate over time.

REVIEW EXERCISES

1. Describe the effect of mA, exposure time, and kVp on film density.

2. Describe the effect of film density and kVp on film contrast.

3. Describe darkroom design requirements.

4. List the chemical components of developer solution, and describe the action of each.

5. List the chemical components of fixer solution, and describe the action of each.

6. List factors that affect the life of processing solutions.

7. Describe manual processing using the time-temperature technique.

8. Describe solution preparation, replenishment, and testing.

9. Describe the coin test.

10. Describe light-leak testing.

11. Describe proper film storage.

12. Define all the terms listed at the end of the Learning Objectives in this chapter.

LEARNING ACTIVITIES

Learning Activity 5-1: The Darkroom

Equipment:

None

Location:

Darkroom

Activity:

Identify and describe the correct use of the following processing equipment:

Manual film processing equipment
Automatic film processing equipment
Lighting/safelighting
View box
Timer
Thermometer
Stepwedge
Film hangers
Film dryer
Solution stirrers

Learning Activity 5-2: Facility Assessment

Equipment:

None

Activity:

Identify local and federal regulations regarding the disposal of processing waste. Evaluate your facility's compliance with these regulations.

Strengths:

Weaknesses:

Recommendations:

Learning Activity 5-3: Solution Change

Equipment:

Concentrated processing solutions
Tank brushes/cleaners
Mild detergent

Location:

Darkroom

Activity:

Following the above guidelines, dispose of the old processing chemicals, clean the processing tanks, and prepare new solutions.

Learning Activity 5-4: Factors which Influence Density and Contrast/Manual Processing

Equipment:

Stepwedge
12, #2 films
6 film racks

Location:

X-ray operatory and darkroom

Activity:

1. Expose 6 stepwedge films as for solution testing. Label 1 to 6.
2. Keeping the PID the same, expose the following films using the stepwedge (change only the indicated settings):

   Film 7: Alter the milliamp setting from the usual (from 10 to 15 mA or from 15 to 10 mA). Label it 7.

Film 8: Increase the exposure time by 20 percent. Label it 8.

Film 9: Decrease the exposure time by 20 percent. Label it 9.

Film 10: Expose at 65 kVp. Label it 10.

Film 11: Expose at 75 kVp. Label it 11.

Film 12: Expose at 90 kVp. Label it 12.

3. Under safelight conditions and labeling the films, process the films as follows:

Films 1, 7, 8, 9, 10, 11, and 12: Use the time-temperature technique developing at 68°F for 4½ minutes, rinse, fix for 10 minutes, wash 20 minutes, and dry. *Save film 6 for* Learning Activity 5-5.

Film 2: Develop at 68°F for 2 minutes. Rinse, fix, and wash as usual.

Film 3: Develop at 68°F for 6 minutes. Rinse, fix, and wash as usual.

Film 4: Develop for 4½ minutes at 60°F. Rinse, fix, and wash as usual.

Film 5: Develop for 4½ minutes at 76°F. Rinse, fix, and wash as usual.

4. Compare the density and scale of contrast of the films with the control film (film 1). Indicate an increase with a plus sign and a decrease with a minus sign.

Exposure/Processing Conditions	Density	Scale of Contrast
Film 1:		
Film 2:		
Film 3:		
Film 4:		
Film 5:		
Film 6:		
Film 7:		
Film 8:		
Film 9:		
Film 10:		
Film 11:		
Film 12:		

5. How does the temperature of the developer affect film density? contrast? Explain.

6. How does developing time affect film density? contrast? Explain.

7. How does milliamperage affect film density? contrast? Explain.

8. How does exposure time affect film density? contrast? Explain.

9. How does kilovoltage affect film density? contrast? Explain.

Learning Activity 5-5: Automatic Processing

Equipment:

Automatic processor
Film 6

Location:

Darkroom

Activity:

1. Follow the manufacturer's directions to prepare the automatic processor. Process film 6.

2. Compare film 6 with film 1. Assess density, contrast, sharpness. Do the images differ in any way? Explain.

3. Assess the advantages and disadvantages of manual and automatic processing:

Manual

Advantages:

Disadvantages:

Automatic

Advantages:

Disadvantages:

Learning Activity 5-6: Automatic Processor Maintenance

Equipment:

Automatic processor
Manufacturer's instruction manual

Location:

Darkroom

Activity:

1. Review the cleaning and maintenance procedures for your automatic processor.
2. Demonstrate the correct procedure for replenishing the solutions (if required).
3. Demonstrate the correct procedure for cleaning the processor.

Learning Activity 5-7: Light-Leak Testing/Safelight Testing

Equipment:

Film
Penny or other coin

Location:

Darkroom

Activity:

1. Close the door, and turn off all the lights.
2. Wait until your eyes adjust to the dark, and then look around the room for areas where you can see white light. Identify such areas and have them repaired.
3. Unwrap the film, place it on the counter, and place the coin on top of it.
4. Turn on the safelight, and wait 5 minutes.
5. Remove the coin, and process the film.
6. Check the film. Does the outline of the coin appear? If so, evaluate your safelighting.

BIBLIOGRAPHY

De Lyre, Wolf R., and Johnson, Orlen N. *Essentials of Dental Radiography for Dental Assistants and Hygienists,* 4th ed. Norwalk, Conn., Appleton and Lange, 1985.

Frommer, Herbert H. *Radiology for Dental Auxiliaries,* 5th ed. St. Louis, C.V. Mosby, 1992.

Goaz, Paul W., and White, Stuart C. *Oral Radiology: Principles and Interpretation,* 2d ed. St. Louis, C.V. Mosby, 1987.

Miles, Dale A., Van Dis, Margot L., et al. *Radiographic Imaging for Dental Auxiliaries.* Philadelphia. W.B. Saunders Company, 1989.

Film Mounting and the Identification of Processing Errors

6

After completing this chapter the student will be able to

1. Correctly position a film during exposure to facilitate mounting.
2. Describe and demonstrate the American Dental Association (ADA) recommended mounting method to correctly mount a full-mouth survey.
3. List general anatomic characteristics that aid mounting.
4. Identify anatomic landmarks used to facilitate mounting, including

   Median palatine suture
   Incisive foramen
   Nasal fossa
   Nasal septum
   Anterior nasal spine
   Junction of the nasal fossa and the maxillary sinus
   Maxillary sinus
   Zygomatic process
   Malar bone
   Zygomatic arch

   Maxillary tuberosity
   Hamular process and notch
   Coronoid process
   Lingual foramen
   Genial tubercle
   Mental ridge
   Nutrient canals
   Mental foramen
   Mandibular canal
   External and internal oblique ridges

5. Identify processing and film handling errors in processed radiographs.
6. Describe and demonstrate the correct procedure for duplicating radiographs.
7. Define the following terms:

   Anatomic landmark
   Duplication

   Mount
   Processing error

I. FILM MOUNTING

A. Mounting Radiographs

To facilitate viewing and interpretation of radiographic surveys, films are placed in cardboard or plastic holders called **mounts.** Opaque materials are preferred because they block the concentrated light used for viewing radiographs and enhance film viewing. Mounts are available for many different variations of full-mouth and bitewing surveys (Fig. 6-1).

Film positioning during exposure can facilitate mounting. When positioned correctly, the convexity of the embossed dot on the dental x-ray film faces the teeth and the radiation source. Always position the dot toward the incisal or occlusal surface when exposing periapical films. This will avoid superimposing the dot on anatomic structures or pathology and will simplify mounting.

(Dot in slot)

The *film positioning in the mount* recommended by the American Dental Association (ADA) is to mount the radiographs as though you were looking into the patient's mouth as in a clinical examination:

☑ The convexity of the embossed dot faces the viewer. The patient's right will be on the viewer's left, and vice versa, just as in a clinical examination.

☐ The teeth should appear in their proper order, i.e., molar view, premolar view, canine, and incisor views. Bitewing placement will vary with different mount designs (Fig. 6-2).

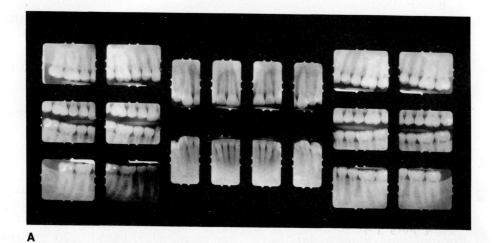

A

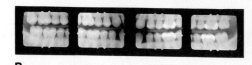

B

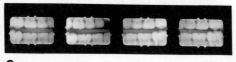

C

Figure 6-1. Various full-mouth survey and bitewing mounts. (**A**) Adult full-mouth survey. (**B**) Adult bitewing survey. (**C**) Pedodontic bitewing survey.

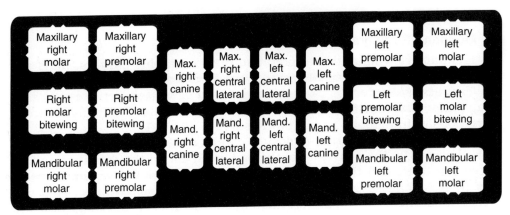

Figure 6-2. Mounting order.

B. Mounting Procedure

1. Wash and thoroughly dry your hands to avoid fingerprints.

2. Touch only the outer edges of the film whenever possible.
   Note: Mount only one set of films at a time to avoid confusion.

3. Use a view box on a clean, dry surface. If the surface is dark, place the films on a white paper for easier identification.

4. Identify anterior, posterior, and bitewing views, and group them together with the embossed dot facing you.

5. Label the mount with the patient's name and the date on which the films were exposed.

6. Mount the bitewing films, and use them to identify restorations and missing teeth that will assist in mounting the other radiographs.

7. Using the anatomic landmarks below and the bitewing radiographs, mount the periapical radiographs.

C. General Guidelines for Mounting

☐ Maxillary anterior teeth are generally larger than their mandibular counterparts (Fig. 6-3A).

☐ Normally, maxillary molars have three roots, while mandibular molars have only two (Fig. 6-3B).

☐ Normally, most roots curve distally (Fig. 6-3C).

☐ The occlusal plane of both arches curves upward. The maxilla is convex, and the mandible is concave (Fig. 6-3D).

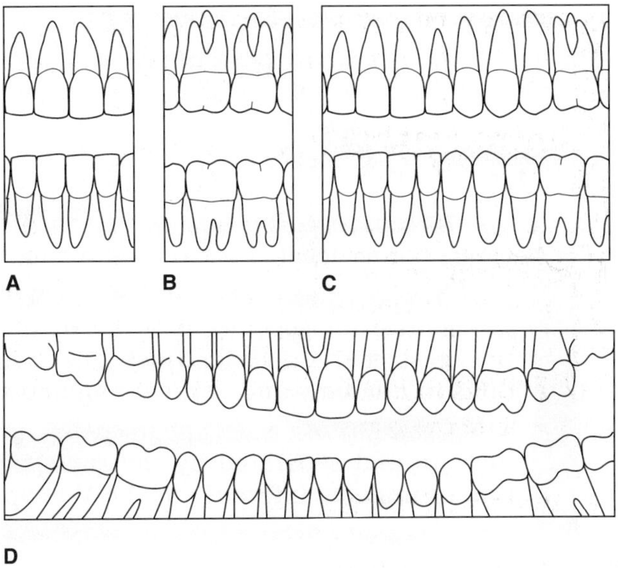

Figure 6-3. **(A)** Maxillary anterior teeth are generally larger than their mandibular counterparts. **(B)** Normally, maxillary molars have three roots, while mandibular molars have only two. **(C)** Normally, most roots curve distally. **(D)** The occlusal plane of both arches curves upward. The maxilla is convex; the mandible is concave.

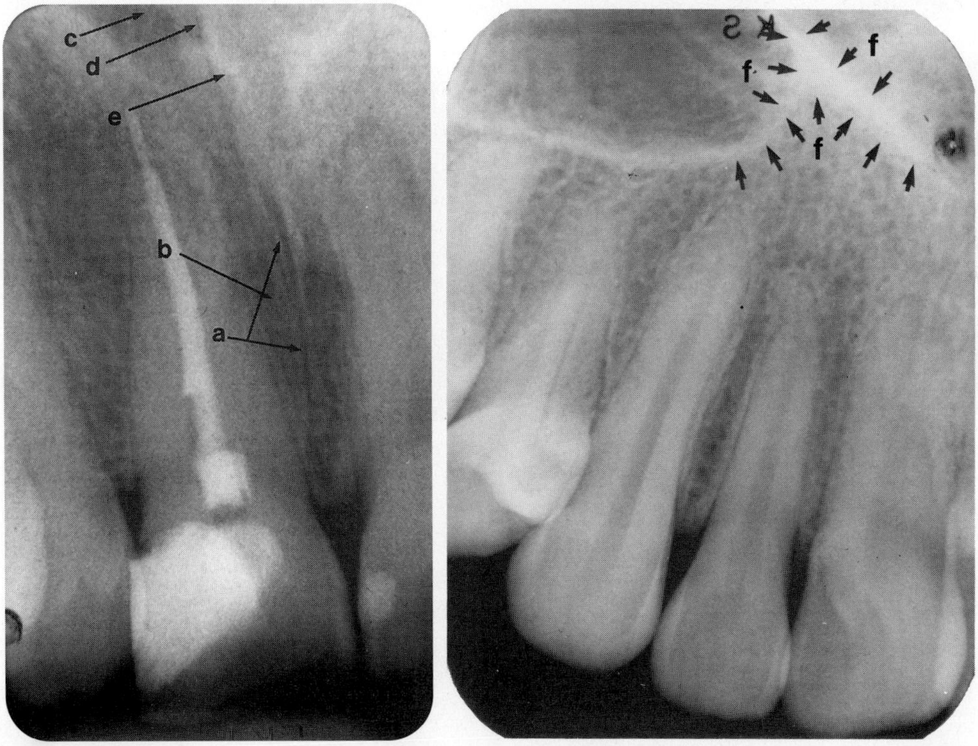

Figure 6-4. Maxillary anterior landmarks. (a) The median palatine suture. (b) The incisive foramen. (c) The nasal fossa. (d) The nasal septum. (e) The anterior nasal spine. (f) The junction of the nasal fossa and the maxillary sinus. (Photo at right from Haring JI, Lind LJ: *Radiographic Interpretation for the Dental Hygienist.* Philadelphia, W.B. Saunders Company, 1993. P. 41.)

The antral Y (upside down) area of max canine

d - radiopaque
e - ″

a - radiolucent
b - ″
c - ″

D. Anatomic Landmarks for Mounting

The following **anatomic landmarks** will assist in identifying the radiographic view and correctly placing the radiographs in the mount:

☐ **Maxillary anterior landmarks** (Fig. 6-4):

- The *median palatine suture* is a thin radiolucent line with a radiopaque border located between the maxillary central incisors.

- The *incisive foramen* is an oval radiolucency between the roots of the central incisors. Its position in the radiograph may vary from the crest of the alveolar ridge to the apical area because of variations in anatomy and vertical angulation.

- The *nasal fossae* are radiolucent areas located above the maxillary incisors and separated by the radiopaque *nasal septum*. The septum terminates inferiorly in the V-shaped *anterior nasal spine*.

- The *junction of the nasal fossa and the maxillary sinus* is a thin

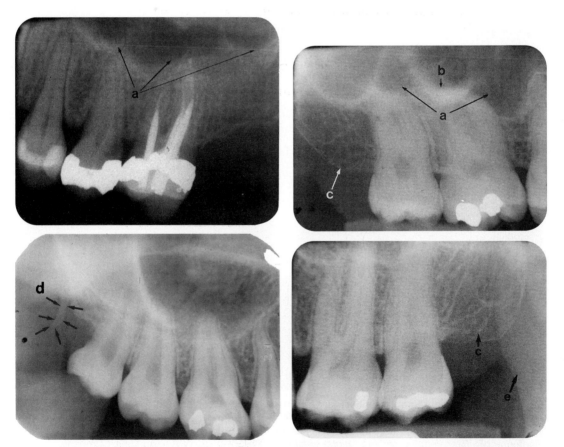

Figure 6-5. Maxillary posterior landmarks. (a) The maxillary sinus. (b) The zygomatic process. (c) The maxillary tuberosity. (d) The hamular process. (e) The coronoid process of the mandible. (Photo, lower left, from Haring JI, Lind LJ: *Radiographic Interpretation for the Dental Hygienist.* Philadelphia, W.B. Saunders Company, 1993. P. 42.

antral Y

radiopaque line that forms a Y above the maxillary canine or first premolar.

❏ **Maxillary posterior landmarks** (Fig. 6-5):

- The maxillary sinus is a large radiolucent area bordered by an irregular radiopaque line located above or superimposed on the apices of the premolars and molars.

- The *zygomatic process* is the U-shaped radiopacity above the roots of the molars. The *malar bone* is the radiopaque band that extends distally from the zygomatic process. Together these bones make up the *zygomatic arch.*

- The *maxillary tuberosity* is a the radiopaque bony protrusion distal to the maxillary molar area.

- The *hamular process* is a bony radiopaque projection distal to the maxillary tuberosity that extends downward. The *hamular notch* is the radiolucent area between the hamular process and the maxillary tuberosity.

- The *coronoid process of the mandible* may be visible as a radiopaque bony projection from the lower distal portion of the radiograph.

❏ **Mandibular anterior landmarks** (Fig. 6-6):

- The *lingual foramen* is the round radiolucency located below the

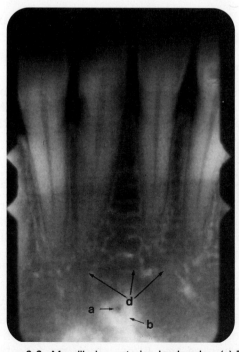
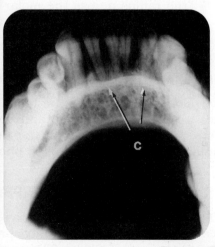

Figure 6-6. Mandibular anterior landmarks. (a) The lingual foramen. (b) The genial tubercle. (c) The mental ridge. (d) Nutrient canals.

Small spines
radiopaque circle

may cover root surfaces of front teeth

(Mentum refers to chin)

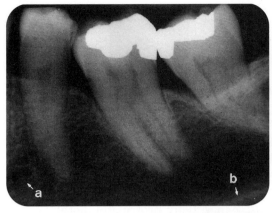
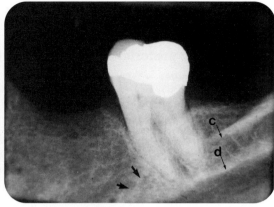

Figure 6-7. Mandibular posterior landmarks. (a) The mental foramen. (b) The mandibular canal. (c) The external oblique ridge. (d) The internal oblique ridge.

mandibular central incisors. The *genial tubercle* is the circular radiopacity that surrounds the lingual foramen.

- The *mental ridge* appears as a radiopaque band extending from below the apex of the canine to the apical area of the incisors.

- *Nutrient canals* may be visible in this region. They appear as vertical radiolucent bands.
  where tiny blood vessels + nerves come thru.

☐ **Mandibular posterior landmarks** (Fig. 6-7):
  where shats are given
- The *mental foramen* is the round radiolucency located near the apices of the mandibular premolars.
  mental nerve

- The *mandibular canal* is the radiolucent band with a thin radiopaque border located below the apices of the posterior teeth.
  nerves come thru

- The *external oblique ridge* is a radiopaque line that extends from the ramus across the molar area. The *internal oblique ridge* (also called the *mylohyoid ridge*) appears as a radiopaque line below the external oblique ridge. *int lower.*

II. COMMON PROCESSING ERRORS

After mounting, examine the films for **processing errors.** Figure 6-8 provides a guide to the cause and correction of many common processing errors. While retakes should be avoided, if an error impairs the radiograph's diagnostic usefulness, it should be retaken.

III. DUPLICATING RADIOGRAPHS

A duplicate set of radiographs may be required for another dentist, insurance requirements, or liability protection. This may be accomplished through the use of film packets containing two films which produce two
Text continued on page 111

Figure 6-8. Common Processing Errors

Error	Cause	Correction
Clear film		
a. totally clear film	Unexposed	Retake
	Film placed in fix before developer	Retake
b. partially clear film 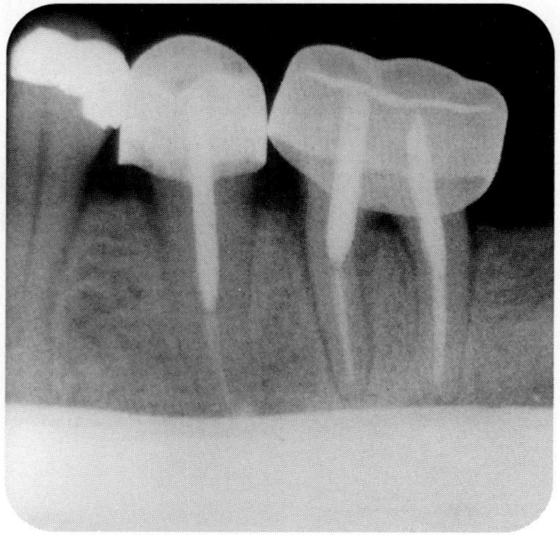	Film not completely immersed in solutions	Always check solution levels prior to processing

Illustration continued on following page

Figure 6-8. *Continued*

Error	Cause	Correction
Light film 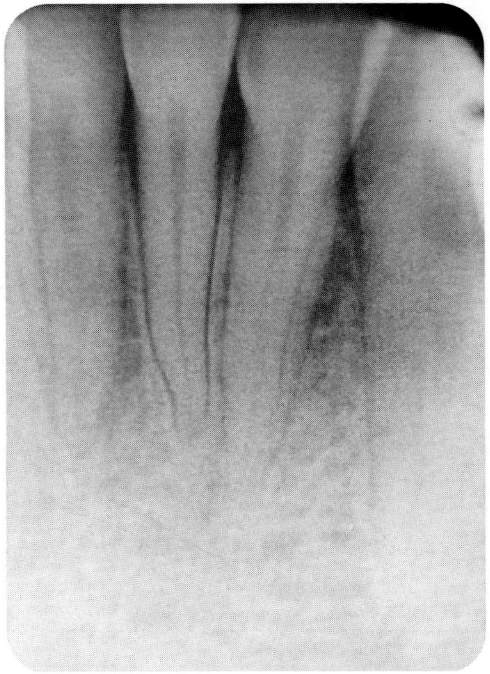	Underexposed	Check exposure time. Increase in 20 percent increments
	Under developed	Check solution temperature (too low?)
		Increase developing time
		Check thermometer and timer accuracy
		Check automatic processor switches, plugs, and thermostat
	Exhausted developer	Change solutions
	Contaminated developer	Change solution

Dark films

Overexposure	Decrease exposure time in 20 percent increments
Overdevelopment	Check solution temperature (too high?)
	Reduce processing time
	Check thermometer and timer accuracy
	Check automatic processor switches, plugs, and thermostat
Exposure to white light	Do coin test/check safelight filter and bulb
	Check for light leaks

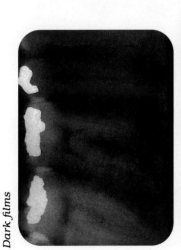

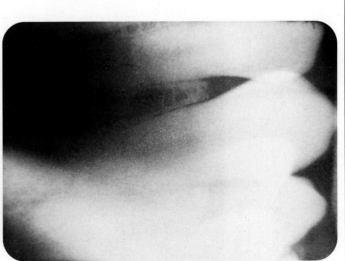

Illustration continued on following page

Figure 6-8. *Continued*

Error	Cause	Correction
Fogged films	Exposure to white light	Do coin test/check safelight filter and bulb
		Check for light leaks
		Do not expose films to white light until they have cleared
	Exposure to heat or radiation	Always keep unexposed films away from exposure area
		Store film at 50 to 70°F
	Outdated film	Check expiration date before using. Rotate film in storage so that oldest will be used first
Yellow/brown stains	Exhausted developer or fixer	Change solutions
	Insufficient time in fix	Refix
	Insufficient washing	Rewash

Streaks

Dirty rollers
Exhausted solutions
Dirty water bath

Clean rollers
Change solutions
Clean water

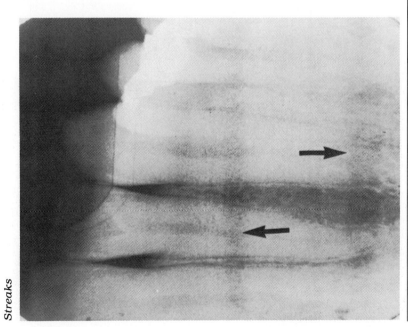

Illustration continued on following page

Figure 6-8. *Continued*

Error	Cause	Correction
Spots 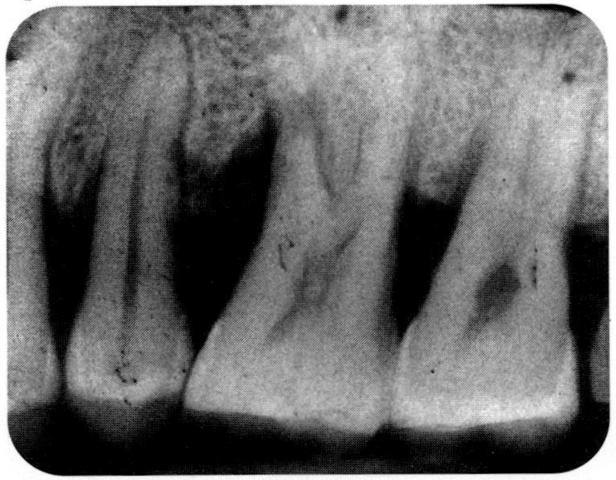	Water/chemical spots	Maintain clean counters
	Dust contamination	
Greenish films	Insufficient fixing	Refix
	Exhausted or contaminated fix	Change solutions
	Films touching during processing	Refix
2 film packets processed without separating		Separate under safelight conditions. Refix

Excessive film bending

Handle films carefully

Static electricity

Black lines

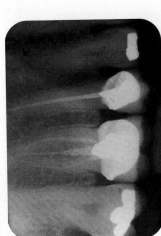 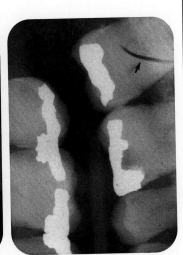

Illustration continued on following page

Figure 6-8. *Continued*

Error	Cause	Correction
White lines	Scratched emulsion	Handle films carefully

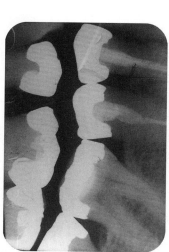

Radiographs for "totally clear film," "fogged film," and "yellow/brown stains" from Haring JI, Lind LJ: *Radiographic Interpretation for the Dental Hygienist*. Philadelphia, W.B. Saunders Company, 1993. Pp. 160, 166, 163, respectively. "Streaks" from Frommer HH: *Radiology for Dental Auxiliaries*, 5th ed. St. Louis, Mosby–Year Book, 1992. P. 118.

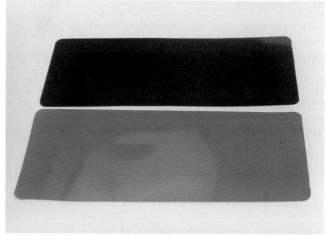

Figure 6-9. Duplicating film. Duplicating film is available in a variety of sizes. This is the 5 × 12 in size used for duplicating full-mouth surveys.

identical radiographs without additional radiation exposure. The **duplication** of existing films is an alternative.

A. Equipment

❏ **Film.** Duplicating film is available in a variety of sizes including 8 × 10 in, 5 × 12 in, and individual periapical size (Fig. 6-9). Its emulsion is on one side only. This side may be identified under safelight conditions as the dull side of the film. Unlike x-ray film, duplicating film becomes lighter as it is exposed to light.

❏ **Duplicator.** Various models and sizes of film duplicators are available. They contain a fluorescent light source under a glass plate on which the films are placed. A cover tightly closes during duplicating. A timer measures duplicating time (Fig. 6-10).

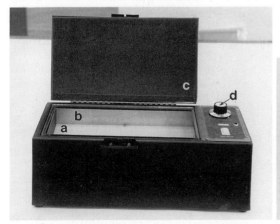
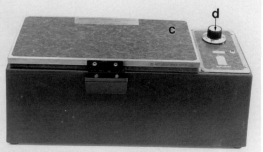

Figure 6-10. Film duplicator. The fluorescent light source (a) is under a glass plate (b) on which the films are placed. The cover (c) tightly closes during duplicating. The timer (d) measures duplicating time.

B. Procedure

Always read the manufacturer's directions for your duplicator carefully before attempting to duplicate films.

Note: Duplicating should be done under safelight conditions.

1. Films to be duplicated should be mounted or placed in film organizers designed for duplicating.

2. Place the film's viewing side up on the glass of the duplicator.

3. Place the duplicating film emulsion side down on top of the films.

4. Close and secure the cover.

5. Set the timer, and duplicate the radiographs.

6. Process as you would any film.

C. The Quality and Appearance of the Duplicate Image

Duplicate radiographs will exhibit less sharpness and a shorter scale of contrast than the original radiographs. Unlike the original radiograph, in the duplicate image, areas exposed to light are clear or light and those not exposed to light are dark. Because of this, density problems in the original films may be corrected in the duplicate radiograph:

❏ To *increase the density* of the duplicate image from that of the original, *decrease the duplicating time.*

❏ To *decrease the density* of the duplicate image from that of the original film, *increase the duplicating time.*

REVIEW EXERCISES

1. How can the film be positioned during exposure to facilitate mounting?

2. Describe the ADA recommended mounting method.

3. List general antomic characteristics that aid mounting.

4. Describe film duplication.

5. Identify the possible cause(s) and correction(s) for the following processing errors:

Error	Cause	Correction
A. Clear film		
(1) Totally clear film		
(2) Partially clear film		
B. Light film		
C. Dark films		
D. Fogged films		

Error	Cause	Correction
E. Yellow/brown stains		
F. Streaks		
G. Spots		
H. Greenish films		
I. Two film packets processed without separating		
J. Black lines		

Error	Cause	Correction
K. White lines		

6. Define all the terms listed at the end of the Learning Objectives in this chapter.

LEARNING ACTIVITIES

Learning Activity 6-1: Identification of Anatomic Landmarks

Equipment:

1 skull

Activity:

Identify the following anatomic landmarks on the skull provided:

Median palatine suture
Incisive foramen
Nasal fossa
Nasal septum
Anterior nasal spine
Junction of the nasal fossa and the maxillary sinus
Maxillary sinus
Zygomatic process
Malar bone
Zygomatic arch
Maxillary tuberosity
Hamular process and notch

Coronoid process
Lingual foramen
Genial tubercle
Mental ridge
Nutrient canals
Mental foramen
Mandibular canal
External and internal oblique ridges

Learning Activity 6-2: Mounting a Full-Mouth Survey

Equipment:

1 exposed and processed full-mouth survey
1 full-mouth survey film mount
1 view box

Activity:

1. Follow the procedures described in this chapter to mount the full-mouth survey.
2. Identify the following anatomic landmarks in the full-mouth survey:
   Median palatine suture
   Incisive foramen
   Nasal fossa
   Nasal septum
   Anterior nasal spine
   Junction of the nasal fossa and the maxillary sinus
   Maxillary sinus
   Zygomatic process
   Malar bone
   Zygomatic arch
   Maxillary tuberosity
   Hamular process and notch
   Coronoid process

Lingual foramen

Genial tubercle

Mental ridge

Nutrient canals

Mental foramen

Mandibular canal

External and internal oblique ridges

3. Identify and list any film processing errors present in the full-mouth survey.

Learning Activity 6-3: Duplicating Radiographs

Equipment:

1 mounted full-mouth survey

Duplicating film

Film duplicator

View box

Location:

Darkroom

Activity:

1. Read the manufacturer's directions for your film duplicator.
2. Follow the directions to duplicate the full-mouth survey.
3. Process the duplicate film.
4. Compare sharpness, contrast, and density of the duplicate and original. Do they differ? How? Explain.

BIBLIOGRAPHY

De Lyre, Wolf R., and Johnson, Orlen N. *Essentials of Dental Radiography for Dental Assistants and Hygienists*, 4th ed. Norwalk, Conn., Appleton and Lange, 1985.

Frommer, Herbert H. *Radiology for Dental Auxiliaries*, 5th ed. St. Louis, C.V. Mosby, 1992.

Goaz, Paul W., and White, Stuart C. *Oral Radiology: Principles and Interpretation,* 2d ed. St. Louis, C.V. Mosby, 1987.

Haring, J. I., and Lind, L. J. *Radiographic Interpretation for the Dental Hygienist.* Philadelphia, W.B. Saunders Company, 1993.

Miles, Dale A., Van Dis, Margot L., et al. *Radiographic Imaging for Dental Auxiliaries.* Philadelphia, W.B. Saunders Company, 1989.

Basic Principles of Shadow Casting and Recording

After completing this chapter the student will be able to

1. List the basic principles of shadow casting and recording.
2. Describe the influence of each principle on the radiographic image.
3. Define the following terms:

Distortion   Radiolucent

Elongation   Radiopaque

Foreshortening   Resolution

Magnification   Sharpness

Opaque   Translucent

Overlapping

I. SHADOW CASTING AND X-RAY IMAGE PRODUCTION

Producing an x-ray image is similar to using light to cast a shadow:

❏ When a shadow is cast, the source of light that creates the shadow may be the sun, a light bulb, or any other light-producing object. The source of radiation that creates the x-ray image lies in a tube within the x-ray tube head.

❏ A shadow is created by an object that blocks light from reaching the surface on which the shadow is cast. Objects that block or absorb light are **opaque.** Some objects, such as windows, do not cast shadows because light passes through them. Objects that do not absorb light are **translucent.** An x-ray image is created by objects that block radiation from reaching the image receptor or x-ray film. Objects that block or absorb radiation, such as teeth, bone, and metal restorations, are **radiopaque.** Most x rays pass through soft tissues such as the gingiva, cheek, and lips. These objects do not create an x-ray image. Objects that do not absorb radiation are **radiolucent.**

❐ A shadow may be recorded on the ground, floor, wall, etc. A radiographic image is recorded on specially prepared film.

II. BASIC PRINCIPLES OF SHADOW CASTING AND RECORDING

In order for a shadow to accurately represent the size and shape of the object that casts it, five principles must be followed. The same principles must be followed if the radiographic image is to accurately depict anatomic structures:

Principle 1: *The source of radiation should be as small as possible.* The source of radiation lies in the x-ray tube at the anode. The *focal spot* is the area of the tungsten target where x rays are created (Fig. 7-1). Its size is determined by the manufacturer of the x-ray machine. To reduce the size of the *effective focal spot*, the tungsten target is placed at a 20 degree angle. The sharpness and resolution of the x-ray image *decrease* as the size of the source of radiation increases.

❐ **Sharpness** is the measure of how clearly small details of the object are reproduced in a radiograph.

❐ **Resolution** is a measure of the ability to see small objects that are close together. The clarity of the radiographic image is the result of the amount of sharpness and resolution in a radiograph.

Principle 2: *The distance from the radiation source to the object should be as long as possible.* The length of the position-indicating device (PID) and the position of the tube within the tube head determine the distance of the radiation source to the object (Fig. 7-2). PIDs vary in length and are classified as short, intermediate, or long by the manufacturer. Because of Principle 2, a PID classified as long should be used.

❐ Sharpness and resolution *increase* as the distance from the tube to the film (TFD) increases. **Magnification,** the increase in the size of the image as compared with the actual size of the object, *decreases* as the tube-film distance increases.

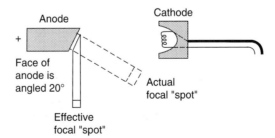

Figure 7-1. Focal spot. The focal spot is the area of the tungsten target where x rays are created. To reduce the size of the effective focal spot and increase sharpness and resolution, the tungsten target is placed at a 20 degree angle.

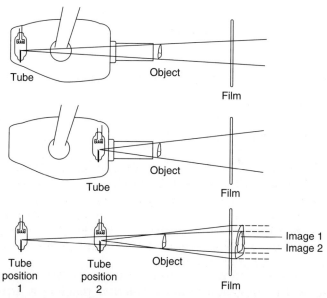

Figure 7-2. Tube-film distance. The length of the position-indicating device (PID) and the position of the tube within the tube head determine the distance of the radiation source to the object. Magnification, the increase in the size of the image as compared with the actual size of the object, decreases as the tube-film distance increases.

Principle 3: *The distance from the object to the recording surface should be as small as possible.* Normal anatomy and patient comfort prevent placing the film directly against the tooth in most areas of the mouth. However, because of this principle, the film should be placed as close to the tooth as possible.

Sharpness and resolution *increase* as distance from the object to the film decreases. Magnification *decreases* as the distance decreases (Fig. 7-3).

Principle 4: *The object and recording surface should be parallel.* When placing the film, two lines should be imagined. The first is a vertical line from the apex to the incisal or occlusal edge of the tooth. The second is a horizontal line from the mesial to distal surfaces. To satisfy Principle 4,

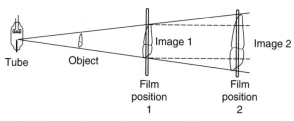

Figure 7-3. The effect of film position on image magnification. The film should be placed as close to the tooth as possible. Sharpness and resolution are improved and magnification is decreased with small tooth to film distances.

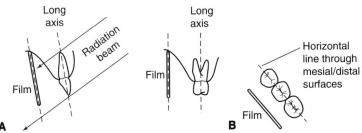

Figure 7-4. Vertical and horizontal parallelism. The tooth and film should be parallel in both vertical and horizontal dimensions. **(A)** Vertically, place the film parallel to a vertical line from the apex to the incisal or occlusal edge of the tooth. **(B)** Horizontally, place it parallel to a horizontal line from the mesial to distal surfaces.

the vertical position of the film must be parallel to the first line. The horizontal position of the film must be parallel to the second line (Fig. 7-4).

☐ If the film is not placed parallel to both lines, points on the tooth closer to the film will exhibit more sharpness and resolution and less magnification than those farther away (see Principle 3). This causes **distortion,** a change in the shape of the image as compared with the object. Distortion *increases* as the relationship between the object and film become less parallel.

Principle 5: *The radiation should strike the object and recording surface at right angles.* The same horizontal and vertical lines as imagined for Principle 4 must be considered. The *vertical angulation* of the x-ray beam should be directed perpendicular to the vertical line. The *horizontal angulation* should be directed perpendicular to the horizontal line (Fig. 7-5). In

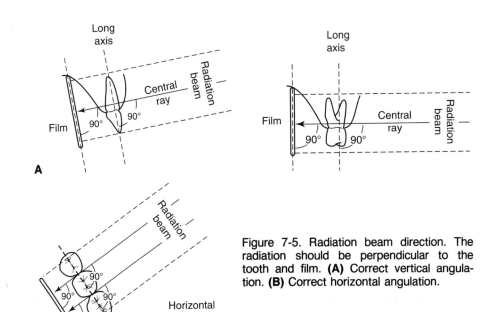

Figure 7-5. Radiation beam direction. The radiation should be perpendicular to the tooth and film. **(A)** Correct vertical angulation. **(B)** Correct horizontal angulation.

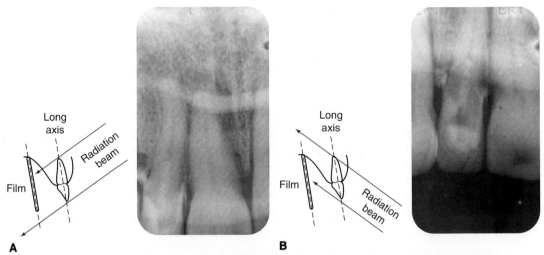

Figure 7-6. Results of incorrect vertical angulation. (A) If the tooth and film are parallel, excessive vertical angulation will project the image incisally (in this case off the film). **(B)** If the tooth and film are parallel, insufficient vertical angulation will project the image apically (in this case off the film).

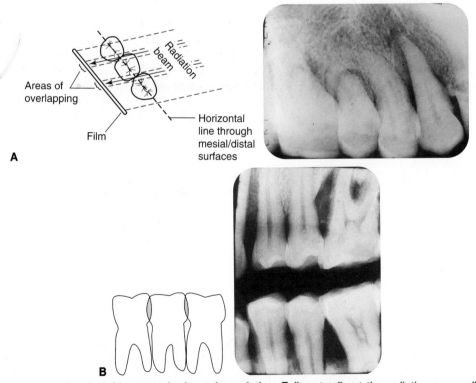

Figure 7-7. Results of incorrect horizontal angulation. Failure to direct the radiation perpendicular to the horizontal line **(A)** will move the image mesially or distally and cause overlapping, the superimposition of the mesial and distal surfaces of adjacent teeth **(B).**

order for the radiation to strike *both* the object and the recording surface at right angles, Principle 4 must be followed.

❏ If the tooth and film are parallel, failure to direct the radiation perpendicular to the vertical line will move the image up or down on the recording surface (Fig. 7-6).

❏ Failure to direct the radiation perpendicular to the horizontal line will move the image mesially or distally and cause **overlapping,** the superimposition of the mesial and distal surfaces of adjacent teeth (Fig. 7-7).

❏ If *both* Principle 4 and Principle 5 are *not* followed and both the film position and radiation beam direction are incorrect, the image of points on the tooth close to the film will exhibit more sharpness and resolu-

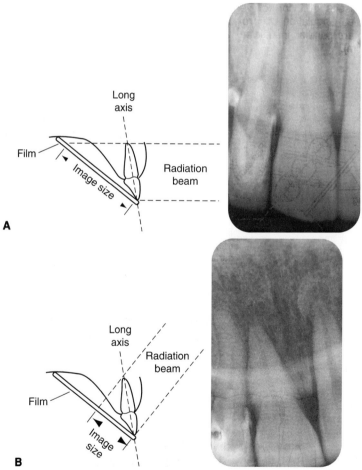

Figure 7-8. Elongation and foreshortening. If the film is not parallel to the tooth and the radiation is not perpendicular to the tooth, **(A)** too little vertical angulation causes the error known as *elongation* (i.e., the image appears longer than the actual length of the object) and **(B)** too much vertical angulation causes *foreshortening* (i.e., the image appears shorter than the actual length of the object).

tion and less magnification than those farther away. In addition, they will exhibit less movement on the film than those farther away. In this case, too little vertical angulation causes the error known as **elongation;** the image appears longer than the actual length of the object (Fig. 7-8A). Too much vertical angulation causes **foreshortening;** the image appears shorter than the actual length of the object (Fig. 7-8B). Elongation and foreshortening are most often seen in vertical angulation errors with the bisecting angle technique (see Chap. 9).

REVIEW EXERCISES

1. List the five principles of shadow casting and recording.

2. What image qualities does each influence?

3. Define all the terms listed at the end of the Learning Objectives in this chapter.

LEARNING ACTIVITIES

Learning Activity 7-1: Principles of Shadow Casting (source of radiation should be as small as possible)

Equipment:

    1 large flashlight
    1 penlight flashlight
    3 paper cups or other solid objects to represent teeth
    1 piece of cardboard approximately 9 × 12 in to represent the film
    a prop to hold the "film" in place
    a 12- or 18-in ruler

Activity:

1. On a tabletop or counter in a darkened room, place the "teeth" in a row so that they are touching.

2. Place the "film" approximately 2 in behind the teeth and parallel to them.

3. Turn on the large flashlight, and direct the light beam perpendicular to the "teeth" and "film." Note the shadow.

4. Keep the "teeth" and "film" in the same position. Change to the penlight, and direct the light beam perpendicular to the teeth and film. Note the shadow.

Questions:

1. How does the shadow created by the large flashlight differ from that created by the penlight

2. Why?

3. State the principle of shadow casting and recording that you have demonstrated.

Learning Activity 7-2: Shadow Casting (distance from source to object should be as long as possible)

Equipment:

Same as those for Learning Activity 7-1 (either or both flashlights may be used).

Activity:

1. Keeping the "film" and "teeth" in the same position, place the flashlight 8 in from the "teeth," and direct the light beam perpendicular to them. Note the shadow.

2. Now move the flashlight 12 in from the "teeth." Note the shadow.

3. Move the flashlight 16 in from the "teeth." Again, note the shadow.

Questions:

1. How does the shadow change as the distance from the light source to the "teeth" increases?
2. Why?
3. State the principle of shadow casting and recording that you have demonstrated.

Learning Activity 7-3: Shadow Casting (distance from object to recording surface should be as small as possible)

Equipment:

Same as those for Learning Activity 7-2.

Activity:

1. Move the flashlight back to the 8-in position.
2. Place the "film" directly behind the "teeth" and parallel to them. Note the shadow.
3. Move the "film" 4 in away from the "teeth," keeping it parallel to them. Note the shadow.
4. Move the "film" 8 in from the "teeth," keeping it parallel to them. Note the shadow.

Questions:

1. How does the shadow change as the distance from the "teeth" to the "film" increases?
2. Why?
3. State the principle of shadow casting and recording that you have demonstrated.

Learning Activity 7-4: Shadow Casting (object and recording surface should be parallel)

Equipment:

Same as those for Learning Activity 7-3.

Activity:

Leaving the "film" in the 8-in position and the light beam in the 16-in position, change the angle of the "film" so that it is no longer parallel with the long axis of the "teeth."

Questions:

1. How does the shadow change?
2. How does the shadow differ on parts of the "film" closer to the "teeth" and those farther away?
3. What is the change in the shadow called?
4. State the principle of shadow casting and recording that you have demonstrated.

Learning Activity 7-5: Shadow Casting (radiation should strike object and recording surface at right angles)

Equipment:

Same as those for Learning Activity 7-4.

Activity:

1. Place the "film" parallel to the "teeth" and approximately 2 in behind them.
2. Holding the flashlight approximately 16 in from the "teeth," make the following adjustments in the vertical angulation of the light beam:

   Direct the beam downward at a 70 degree angle to the tooth and film (+70).

Direct it downward at a 45 degree angle (+45).

Direct it upward at a 70 degree angle (−70).

Direct it upward at a 45 degree angle (−45)

Questions:

1. How does the shadow change as you alter the downward (positive) vertical angulation of the light beam?
2. How does the shadow change as you alter the upward (negative) vertical angulation of the light beam?
3. Why do the preceding changes occur?
4. What are these changes in the shadow called?
5. State the principle of shadow casting and recording that you have demonstrated.

Learning Activity 7-6: Shadow Casting (elongation and foreshortening)

Equipment:

Same as those for Learning Activity 7-5.

Activity:

Change the angle of the "film" so that it is no longer parallel to the long axis of the "teeth" by placing it against the top of the "teeth" and 4 in away at the bottom of the "teeth." Repeat step 2 of Learning Activity 7-5.

Questions:

1. How do the shadow changes differ from those in the preceding exercise?
2. Why?
3. State the principles of shadow casting and recording that you have demonstrated.

Learning Activity 7-7: Shadow Casting (overlapping)

Equipment:

Same as those for Learning Activity 7-6.

Activity:

1. Place a ruler on top of the "teeth" so that it extends from the middle of the "mesial" surface of one "tooth" to the middle of the "distal" surface of the third "tooth."
2. Place the film approximately 2 in behind the "film" and parallel to the ruler as well as the long axis of the "teeth."
3. Holding the flashlight approximately 16 in from the "teeth," make the following adjustments in the horizontal angulation of the light beam:

   Direct the light beam perpendicular to the ruler and the "film."

   Change the horizontal angulation of the light beam 20 degrees to the "mesial."

   Change the horizontal angulation 45 degrees to the "mesial."

   From the original position of the light beam, change the horizontal angulation 20 degrees to the "distal."

   Now change the horizontal angulation 45 degrees to the "distal."

Questions:

1. How does the shadow change as the horizontal angulation moves mesially?
2. How does the shadow change as the horizontal angulation moves distally?
3. Why do these changes occur?
4. State the principle of shadow casting and recording that you have demonstrated.

Learning Activity 7-8: Shadow Casting (object and recording surface should be parallel)

Equipment:

Same as those for Learning Activity 7-7.

Activity:

1. Using the same setup as in Learning Activity 7-7, adjust the position of the "film" so that it is no longer parallel to the ruler.
2. Repeat Activity 3 of Learning Activity 7-7.

Questions:

1. How do the shadow changes differ from those in the preceding exercise?
2. Why?
3. State the principles of shadow casting and recording that you have demonstrated.

BIBLIOGRAPHY

De Lyre, Wolf R., and Johnson, Orlon N. *Essentials of Dental Radiography.* Philadelphia, Prentice-Hall, 1985.

Goaz, Paul W., and White, Stuart C. *Oral Radiology: Principles and Interpretation.* St. Louis, C.V. Mosby, 1987.

The Parallel Technique

8

LEARNING OBJECTIVES

After completing this chapter the student will be able to

1. List the basic principles of the parallel technique.
2. Compare the basic principles of the parallel technique with those of shadow casting and recording.
3. Demonstrate correct film placement and radiation beam direction for the parallel technique on the DXTTR trainer using

   The Rinn instrument.

   The Precision instrument.

   Stabe film holders.
4. Expose full-mouth surveys on the DXTTR trainer with the parallel technique using

   The Rinn instrument.

   The Precision instrument.

   Stabe film holders.
5. Correctly identify the following errors in technique in exposed radiographs:

   Incorrect packet placement

   Cone cut

   Incorrect vertical angulation: excessive, insufficient

   Incorrect horizontal angulation
6. Define the following terms:

   Adjacent   Long axis

   Cone cut   Superimposition

better

The two methods used to expose periapical radiographs are the *parallel* and the *bisecting-angle techniques.* Of these, the parallel technique is preferred because it produces images exhibiting less distortion than those produced by the bisecting-angle technique. To understand why this is true, the basic principles of the parallel technique as well as those of shadow casting and recording must be understood.

I. BASIC PRINCIPLES OF THE PARALLEL TECHNIQUE

A. Packet Placement

The film packet is placed parallel to the teeth to be examined. The film should extend no more than ⅛ to ¼ in beyond the incisal or occlusal edge of the teeth. When placing the film, two lines should be imagined:

❏ The first is a vertical line from the apex to the incisal or occlusal edge of the tooth, which is called the **long axis.** The vertical position of the film must be parallel to this line (see Fig. 7-4A).

❏ The second is a line drawn through the mesial and distal surfaces of the teeth to be examined. The horizontal position of the film must be parallel to this line (see Fig. 7-4B).

In most areas of the mouth, the film must be positioned away from the teeth being examined in order to achieve parallel placement. Failure to place the film parallel to both lines results in distortion. Those areas of the tooth which are farther away from the film will be magnified and will exhibit less sharpness and resolution than those closer to the film.

B. Direction of the X-Ray Beam

The radiation should be perpendicular to the tooth and film.

❏ The *vertical angulation* should be directed perpendicular to the film and the long axis of the tooth (see Fig. 7-5A).
  • Excessive vertical angulation (V+) moves the x-ray image occlusally on the film, demonstrating more apical anatomy. Insufficient vertical angulation (V−) moves the image apically on the film, which may result in inadequate apical coverage (see Fig. 7-6).

❏ The *horizontal angulation* should be directed perpendicular to the line drawn from mesial to distal aspects of the teeth and through the interproximal spaces (see Fig. 7-5B).
  • Failure to do so results in the **superimposition** of proximal surfaces of **adjacent** teeth called *overlapping.* The x-ray image will move mesially if the radiation is directed too much to the mesial and will move distally if the radiation is directed too much to the distal (Fig. 8-1; see also Fig. 7-7).

❏ *Center the film* within the PID.
  • Failure to center the film within the PID results in the technical error called **cone cut.** No image is created in those areas of the film which are not within the PID because they are not exposed to

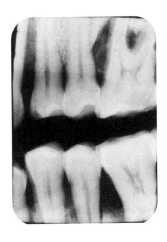

Figure 8-1. Overlapping. Failure to direct the radiation through the interproximal spaces results in the superimposition of proximal surfaces of adjacent teeth called *overlapping.* The x-ray image will move mesially if the radiation is directed too much to the mesial and will move distally if the radiation is directed too much to the distal.

radiation. The border of a cone cut may be round or rectangular depending on the shape of the PID (Fig. 8-2).

C. PID Length

A long PID creates a sharper, less magnified image regardless of the technique used. With the parallel technique, a long cone must be used because, in most areas of the mouth, the film is positioned away from the teeth being examined (see Fig. 7-2).   *8"acceptable — 12" or 16" better choice*

less than 8" cannot do || teching

☐ Sharpness and resolution in the image decrease and magnification increases as the distance from the tooth to the film increases.

☐ A long PID increases the sharpness and resolution and decreases the magnification in the image and, therefore, counteracts the effects of positioning the film at a distance from the teeth.

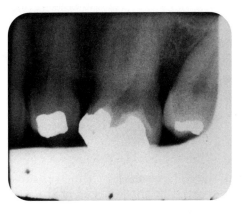

Figure 8-2. Cone cut. Failure to center the film within the PID results in the technical error called *cone cut.* No image is created in those areas of the film which are not within the PID because they are not exposed to radiation. The border of a cone cut may be round or rectangular depending on the shape of the PID.

II. THE PARALLEL TECHNIQUE AND THE BASIC PRINCIPLES OF SHADOW CASTING AND RECORDING COMPARED

As detailed in Chapter 7, the basic principles of shadow casting and recording must be followed in order for the radiographic image to accurately represent dental structures. The following comparison of the basic principles of shadow casting with those of the parallel technique will demonstrate why the parallel technique is preferred.

Principle 1

The source of radiation should be as small as possible.

Parallel Technique

The source of radiation lies within the x-ray tube. Its size is determined by the manufacturer (see Fig. 7-1).

Principle satisfied? ___✓___ Yes _____ No

Principle 2

The distance from the radiation source to the object should be as long as possible.

The sharpness and resolution of the image increases with the use of a long PID. Magnification of the image decreases with the use of a long PID (see Fig. 7-2).

Parallel Technique

A long PID is always used with the parallel technique.

Principle satisfied? ___✓___ Yes _____ No

Principle 3

The distance from the object to the recording surface should be as small as possible.

Sharpness and resolution are best and there is less magnification of the image when the film is close to the tooth (see Fig. 7-3).

Parallel Technique

In most areas of the mouth, the film must be positioned away from the teeth being examined in order to achieve parallel placement.

one principle paralleling
Cannot do !.

Principle satisfied? _____ Yes ___✓___ No

Principle 4

The object and recording surface should be parallel.

Parallel Technique

The film is positioned parallel to the teeth being examined.

If the tooth and film are parallel, all points on the x-ray image will exhibit equal sharpness, resolution, and magnification (see Fig. 7-4).

Principle satisfied? ___✓___ Yes _____ No

Principle 5   *Parallel Technique*

The radiation should strike the object and recording surface at right angles.

The radiation is directed at right angles to the teeth and the film.

Image distortion occurs if the radiation is not directed at right angles to the tooth and film (see Figs. 7-6, 7-7, and 7-8).

Principle satisfied? ___✓___ Yes _____ No

The parallel technique satisfies all the principles of shadow casting and recording with the exception of Principle 3. Failure to follow this principle decreases the sharpness and resolution and increases the magnification of the x-ray image. For this reason, a long PID must always be used with the parallel technique. Use of a long PID increases sharpness and resolution, decreases magnification, and counteracts the effects of a long object-film distance.

Because it satisfies most of the principles of shadow casting and recording, the parallel technique, when used correctly, produces sharp radiographic images that accurately represent the size, shape, and location of anatomic structures.

III. THE PARALLEL TECHNIQUE WITH FILM HOLDERS/AIMING DEVICES

In order to achieve proper film placement, it is necessary to use film holders (see Chap. 3). Film holders attached to aiming devices assist the operator in correctly directing the x-ray beam and reduce the number of retakes due to technical errors. Film holders and aiming devices that provide or may be used with rectangular collimation allow the best reduction in patient exposure by minimizing retakes and reducing the area exposed to radiation.

A. The Stabe Film Holder

This film holder may be used for both anterior and posterior views.

❑ For anterior views, size 0 or 1 film is positioned with its longest side in a vertical position (Fig. 8-3).

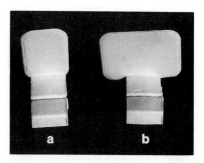

Figure 8-3. Film position in the Stabe film holder for anterior (a) and posterior (b) views. (Courtesy of Rinn Corporation, Elgin, Illinois.)

❏ For posterior adult views, size 2 film is positioned with its longest side in a horizontal position (see Fig. 8-3).

❏ The film and holder are placed behind and parallel to the teeth to be examined. The bite block should rest against the incisal or occlusal edge of the teeth. The patient then closes his or her mouth to hold the film in place (Fig. 8-4).

❏ The vertical angulation should be directed perpendicular to the long axis of the teeth and the film. The visible end of the bite block, which

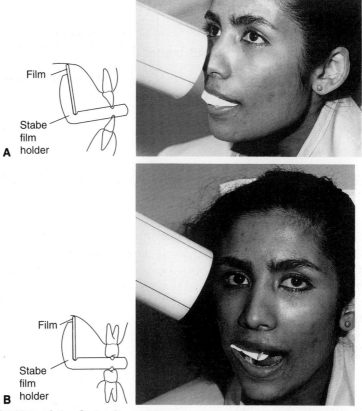

Figure 8-4. Position of the Stabe film holder for anterior **(A)** and posterior **(B)** views. (Courtesy of Rinn Corporation, Elgin, Illinois.)

is parallel to the film, may be used to assist in correctly directing the radiation beam.

❑ The horizontal angulation should be directed through the interproximal spaces and perpendicular to a line that extends from mesial to distal aspects of the teeth to be examined. The bite block may be used again as a guide.

B. The Precision Instrument

This film holder/aiming device also provides rectangular collimation when used with a round, open-ended PID. Three Precision Instruments are needed for full mouth periapicals:

❑ The anterior instrument holds size 0 or 1 film in a vertical position.

❑ Two posterior instruments, one for the upper right and lower left and one for the upper left and lower right, hold size 2 film in a horizontal position.

❑ A plastic bite block slides over the arm of each instrument and allows the patient to hold the instrument securely.

❑ The instrument is placed behind and parallel to the teeth to be examined. The bite block should be against the occlusal or incisal edge (Fig. 8-5).

❑ The PID is positioned so that all points on its edge are equidistant from the aiming circle (Fig. 8-6).

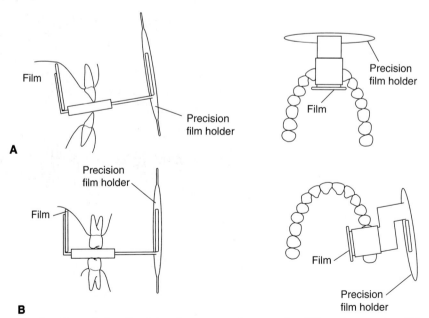

Figure 8-5. Position of the Precision instrument for anterior **(A)** and posterior **(B)** views. (Courtesy of Masel Orthodontics, Bristol, Pennsylvania.)

Figure 8-6. Precision instrument. The PID is positioned so that all points on its edge are equidistant from the aiming circle. (Courtesy of Masel Orthodontics, Bristol, Pennsylvania.)

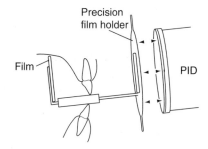

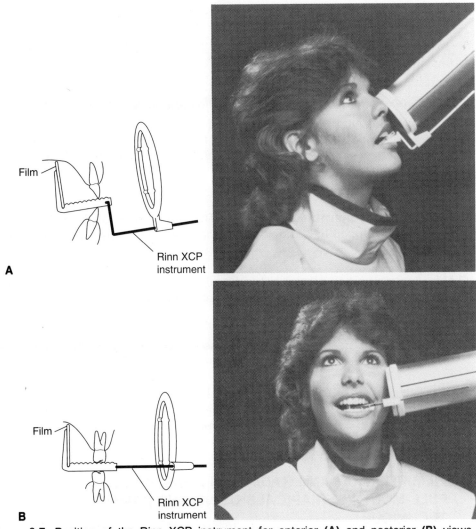

Figure 8-7. Position of the Rinn XCP instrument for anterior **(A)** and posterior **(B)** views. (Courtesy of Rinn Corporation, Elgin, Illinois.)

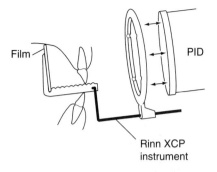

Figure 8-8. Rinn instrument. The PID is positioned so that all points on its edge are equidistant from the aiming ring. (Courtesy of Rinn Corporation, Elgin, Illinois.)

Figure 8-9. The corners of a rectangular PID should be equidistant from the notches on the aiming ring. (Courtesy of Rinn Corporation, Elgin, Illinois.)

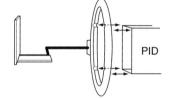

C. The Rinn XCP (Extension Cone Paralleling) Instrument

This device may be used with a rectangular PID or with rectangular collimators which snap on to the aiming ring (see Fig. 3-20). Three instruments are needed for full mouth periapicals.

☐ The anterior instrument holds size 0 or 1 film in a vertical position.

☐ Two posterior instruments, one for the upper right and lower left and one for the upper left and lower right, hold size 2 film in a horizontal position.

☐ The instrument is placed behind and parallel to the teeth to be examined. The bite block should be against the occlusal or incisal edge (Fig. 8-7).

☐ If a round PID is used, the PID is positioned so that all points on its edge are equidistant from the aiming circle (Fig. 8-8).

☐ If a rectangular PID is used, it must be turned so that its longest sides are vertical for anterior views and horizontal for posterior views. The corners of the PID must be equidistant from the notches on the aiming ring (Fig. 8-9).

IV. FILM POSITION AND RADIATION BEAM DIRECTION FOR FULL-MOUTH PERIAPICALS USING THE PARALLEL TECHNIQUE

The views shown in Figs. 8-10 through 8-17 are exposed on the right and left sides for a total of 16 periapical views. The number of films and film sizes in the full-mouth survey will vary with the dentist's training and preference. Views of all tooth-bearing areas must be exposed.

Text continued on page 145

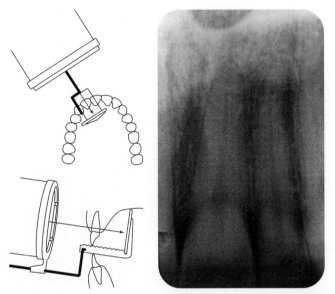

Figure 8-10. Film placement and radiation beam direction for the maxillary central lateral view. (Courtesy of Rinn Corporation, Elgin, Illinois.)

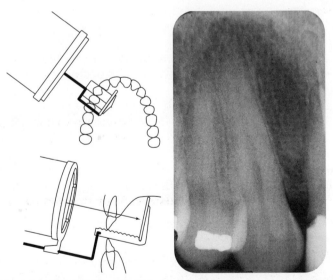

Figure 8-11. Film placement and radiation beam direction for the maxillary canine view. (Courtesy of Rinn Corporation, Elgin, Illinois.)

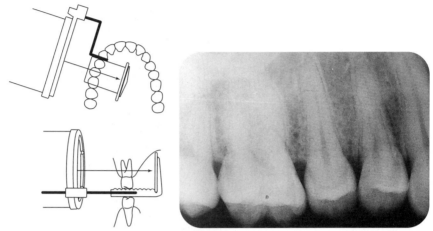

Figure 8-12. Film placement and radiation beam direction for the maxillary premolar view. (Courtesy of Rinn Corporation, Elgin, Illinois.)

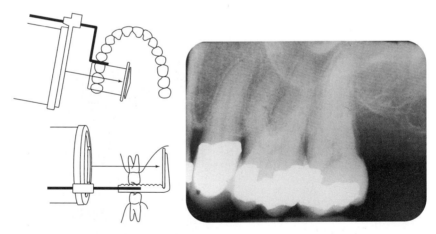

Figure 8-13. Film placement and radiation beam direction for the maxillary molar view. (Courtesy of Rinn Corporation, Elgin, Illinois.)

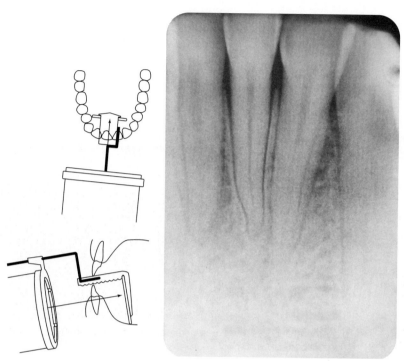

Figure 8-14. Film placement and radiation beam direction for the mandibular central lateral view. (Courtesy of Rinn Corporation, Elgin, Illinois.)

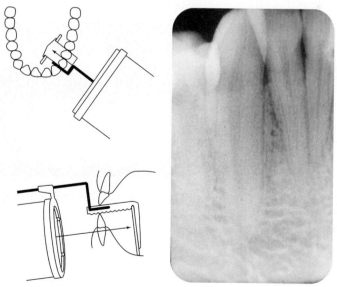

Figure 8-15. Film placement and radiation beam direction for the mandibular canine view. (Courtesy of Rinn Corporation, Elgin, Illinois.)

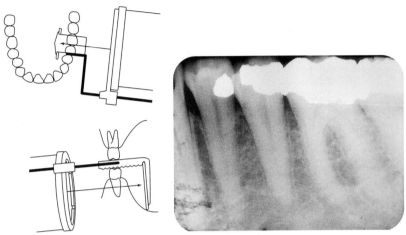

Figure 8-16. Film placement and radiation beam direction for the mandibular premolar view. (Courtesy of Rinn Corporation, Elgin, Illinois.)

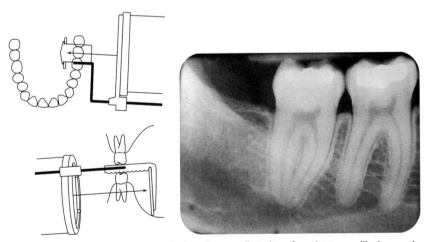

Figure 8-17. Film placement and radiation beam direction for the mandibular molar view. (Courtesy of Rinn Corporation, Elgin, Illinois.)

1. List the basic principles of the parallel technique.

2. List the basic principles of shadow casting and recording.

3. Compare the basic principles of the parallel technique with those of shadow casting and recording.

4. Define all the terms listed at the end of the Learning Objectives in this chapter.

══**LEARNING ACTIVITIES**════

Learning Activity 8-1: Effects of Angulation and Film Positioning Changes

Equipment:

> 7 size 2 films
> Assembled Rinn XCP posterior film holder
> Round open-ended PID (if available)
> DXTTR trainer
> Film mounts

Location:

X-ray operatory and darkroom

Activity:

Seven exposures will be made of the maxillary premolar view (left or right), altering the vertical and horizontal angulation and film placement. When processed, these films will demonstrate the effect of vertical and horizontal radiation errors on films exposed with the parallel technique.

Exposure 1:
1. Using the XCP film holder and number 2 film, correctly place the film for a premolar view:

   Behind and parallel to the premolars.

   Bite block against the occlusal edges.
2. Direct the radiation perpendicular to the tooth and film by aligning the PID with the aiming ring. Make sure that all points on the PID are equidistant from the aiming ring. Note the vertical angulation.
3. Expose the film. Label it Exposure 1.

Exposure 2:
1. Place the film exactly as for Exposure 1.
2. Keeping the top of the PID against the top of the aiming ring, increase the vertical angulation by 10 degrees.
3. Expose the film. Label it PV+.

Exposure 3:
1. Place the film exactly as for Exposure 1.
2. Keeping the PID against the bottom of the aiming ring, decrease the vertical angulation by 10 degrees.
3. Expose the film. Label it PV−.

Exposure 4:
1. Place the film exactly as for Exposure 1.
2. Align the PID so that its right side touches the right side of the aiming ring. The left side of the PID should be 1 in away from the left side of the aiming ring.
3. Expose the film. Label it PHR.

Exposure 5:
1. Place the film exactly as for Exposure 1.
2. Align the PID so that its left side touches the left side of the aiming ring. The right side should be 1 in away from the right side of the aiming ring.
3. Expose the film. Label it PHL.

Exposure 6:
1. Place the film in a nonparallel position by placing the lower edge of the film closer to the long axis than the upper edge.

2. Align the PID as in Exposure 1.

3. Expose the film. Label it PV.

Exposure 7:
1. Place the film in a nonparallel position by placing the distal edge of the film closer to the teeth than the mesial edge.

2. Align the PID as in Exposure 1.

3. Expose the film. Label it PH.

Processing:
Process, mount, and label the films in the order they were taken. (Save these films for Learning Activity 9-2.)

Questions:

1. Compare the x-ray images in films 1, V+, and V−. How does the image change? Why?

2. Compare the x-ray images in films 1, PHR, and PHL. How does the image change? Why?

3. Compare the x-ray images in films 1, PV, and PH. How does the image change? Why?

Learning Activity 8-2: The Rinn XCP Instrument

Equipment:

8 size 0 or 1 films, 8 size 2 films

Rinn XCP setup for full-mouth x-rays

DXTTR trainer

Full-mouth survey mounts

Location:

X-ray operatory and darkroom

Activity:

1. Expose all periapical views contained in an adult full-mouth survey using the parallel technique.

2. Process and mount the films.

Evaluation:

1. Examine the films for the following errors:

   Incorrect vertical angulation (V+ or V−).

   Incorrect horizontal angulation (H).

   Incorrect packet placement (P):

   > Is there distortion caused by lack of parallelism between the teeth and film?

   > Do the correct teeth appear in each film?

   Cone cut.

2. List each film that contains an error, and state the cause of the error and its correction. Circle any films that are diagnostically unacceptable and should be retaken.

Film	Error	Cause	Correction

Learning Activity 8-3: The Stabe Film Holder

Equipment:

8 size 0 or 1 films, 8 size 2 films

Stabe film holder

DXTTR trainer

Full-mouth survey mount

Location:

X-ray operatory and darkroom

Activity:

1. Expose all periapical views contained in an adult full-mouth survey using the parallel technique.
2. Process and mount the films.

Evaluation:

1. Examine the films for the following errors:

   Incorrect vertical angulation (V+ or V−).

   Incorrect horizontal angulation (H).

   Incorrect packet placement (P):

   Is there distortion caused by lack of parallelism between the teeth and film?

   Do the correct teeth appear in each film?

   Cone cut.

2. List each film that contains an error, and state the cause of the error and its correction. Circle any films that are diagnostically unacceptable and should be retaken.

Film	Error	Cause	Correction

Learning Activity 8-4: The Precision Instrument

Equipment:

8 size 0 or 1 films, 8 size 2 films.
Precision instrument
DXTTR trainer
Full-mouth survey mount

Location:

X-ray operatory and darkroom

Activity:

1. Expose all periapical views contained in an adult full-mouth survey using the parallel technique.
2. Process and mount the films.

Evaluation:

1. Examine the films for the following errors:
   Incorrect vertical angulation (V+ or V−).
   Incorrect horizontal angulation (H).
   Incorrect packet placement (P):
     Is there distortion caused by lack of parallelism between the teeth and film?
     Do the correct teeth appear in each film?
   Cone cut.
2. List each film that contains an error, and state the cause of the error and its correction. Circle any films that are diagnostically unacceptable and should be retaken.

Film	Error	Cause	Correction

Film	Error	Cause	Correction

BIBLIOGRAPHY

Frommer, Herbert H. *Radiology for Dental Auxiliaries,* 5th ed. St. Louis, Mosby–Year Book, 1992.

Goaz, Paul G., and White, Stuart C. *Oral Radiography: Principles and Interpretation.* St. Louis, C.V. Mosby, 1989.

Rinn Corporation. *Intraoral Radiography with Rinn XCP/BAI Instruments.* Elgin, Ill., Rinn Corp., 1989.

The Bisecting-Angle Technique

9

LEARNING OBJECTIVES

After completing this chapter the student will be able to

1. List the basic principles of the bisecting-angle technique.

2. Compare the basic principles of the bisecting-angle technique with those of shadow casting and recording and the parallel technique.

3. Demonstrate correct film placement and radiation beam direction for the bisecting-angle technique on the DXTTR trainer using

   The Rinn BAI

   Stabe film holders

4. Expose full-mouth surveys on the DXTRR trainer with the bisecting angle technique using

   The Rinn BAI

   Stabe film holders

5. Correctly identify the following errors in technique in exposed radiographs:

   Incorrect packet placement

   Cone cut

   Incorrect vertical angulation: excessive, insufficient

   Incorrect horizontal angulation

6. Define the following term:

   Bisector

Prior to the advent of film holders, the bisecting-angle technique was used routinely to expose intraoral radiographs. The technique is still used in situations where parallel film placement is impossible due to intraoral anatomy. Distortion is impossible to avoid in images created by the bisecting-angle technique because of the principles of film placement and radiation beam direction used in this technique.

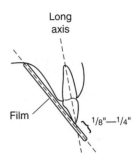

Figure 9-1. Packet placement for the bisecting-angle technique. The film is placed against the incisal or occlusal edge of the teeth to be examined with no more than ⅛ to ¼ in extending beyond the edge. The film diverges from the tooth as it extends vertically to the palate or the floor of the mouth, forming an angle between the long axis of the tooth and the film.

I. THE BASIC PRINCIPLES OF THE BISECTING-ANGLE TECHNIQUE

A. Packet Placement

The film is placed against the incisal or occlusal edge of the teeth to be examined with no more than ⅛ to ¼ in extending beyond the edge. From this point, the film diverges from the tooth as it extends vertically to the palate or the floor of the mouth. In this manner, an angle is formed between the long axis of the tooth and the film (Fig. 9-1). As with the parallel technique, the film is parallel to an imaginery line through the mesial and distal surfaces of the teeth (see Fig. 7-4B).

B. Direction of the X-ray Beam

The radiation should be perpendicular to an imaginery line called the **bisector** which divides the angle formed by the tooth and film into two equal angles (Fig. 9-2).

❑ The *vertical angulation* should be directed perpendicular to the bisector of the angle formed by the tooth and film. Excessive vertical angulation (V+) causes *foreshortening* of the image; it appears shorter than its actual size (see Fig. 7-8B). Insufficient vertical angulation (V−) causes *elongation* of the image; it appears longer than its actual size (see Fig. 7-8A).

❑ The *horizontal angulation* should be directed perpendicular to the imaginery line that extends from mesial to distal aspects of the teeth

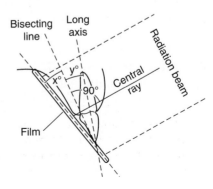

Figure 9-2. Radiation beam direction for the bisecting-angle technique. The radiation is directed perpendicular to the bisector of the angle formed by the long axis of the tooth and the film.

and through the interproximal spaces (see Fig. 7-5*B*). As with the parallel technique, incorrect horizontal angulation causes overlapping and movement of the image mesially or distally depending on the direction of the x-ray beam (see Fig. 7-7).

❑ *Center the film within the PID.* Failure to center the film within the PID results in the technical error called *cone cut.* No image is created in those areas of the film which are not within the PID because they are not exposed to radiation. The border of a cone cut may be round or rectangular depending on the shape of the PID (see Fig. 8-2).

C. PID Length

Either a long or short PID may be used. Sharpness and resolution will be improved with the use of a long PID (see Fig. 7-2).

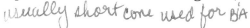
usually short cone used for B/A

II. THE BISECTING-ANGLE TECHNIQUE AND THE BASIC PRINCIPLES OF SHADOW CASTING AND RECORDING COMPARED

As previously described, the basic principles of shadow casting and recording must be followed in order for the x-ray image to accurately represent dental structures. The following comparison of the basic principles of shadow casting with those of the bisecting-angle technique will demonstrate why the parallel technique is preferred:

Principle 1

The source of radiation should be as small as possible.

Bisecting-Angle Technique

The source of radiation lies within the x-ray tube. Its size is determined by the manufacturer.

Principle satisfied?____✓____Yes_____No

Principle 2

The distance from the radiation source to the object should be as long as possible.

The sharpness and resolution of the image increase with use of a long PID. Magnification of the image decreases with use of a long PID.

Bisecting-Angle Technique

A long or short PID may be used with the bisecting-angle technique. While a long PID produces a better x-ray image, it is sometimes difficult to position at the angles required by this technique.

Principle satisfied?_____Yes_____No____✓____Maybe

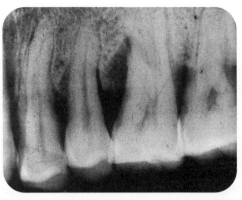 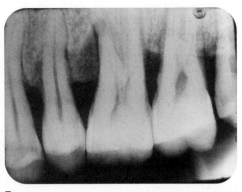

A   **B**

Figure 9-3. Distortion caused by lack of parallelism between the tooth and the film. Both films demonstrate two views of the maxillary premolar area. Film **A** was taken using the parallel technique; film **B**, using the bisecting-angle technique. Note the distortion of the image present in film **B**.

Principle 3

The distance from the object to the recording surface should be as small as possible.

Sharpness and resolution are best and there is less magnification of the image when the film is close to the tooth.

Bisecting-Angle Technique

The film is close to the tooth at the occlusal or incisal edge and diverges from this point to form an angle with the long axis of the tooth. The image of the crown is therefore more accurate than that of the root and apex. This produces distortion of the x-ray image (Fig. 9-3).

proportional distortion

Principle satisfied?_____Yes_____No__✓__Partially

Principle 4

The object and recording surface should be parallel.

If the tooth and film are parallel, all points on the x-ray image will exhibit equal sharpness, resolution, and magnification.

Bisecting-Angle Technique

The bisecting-angle positions the film at an angle to the tooth. Because of this, the image is distorted, as described in Principle 3 (see Fig. 9-3).

Principle satisfied?_____Yes__✓__No

Principle 5

The radiation should strike the object and recording surface at right angles.

Bisecting-Angle Technique

Since the tooth and film meet to form an angle, the radiation cannot be directed perpendicular to both.

Image distortion occurs if the radiation is not directed at right angles to the tooth and film.

Instead, it is directed perpendicular to the bisector of the angle formed by the tooth and film. Because of the direction of the radiation beam, points on the buccal surfaces appear to be positioned more coronally than their lingual counterparts creating image distortion.

Principle satisfied?_____Yes___✓__No

The bisecting-angle technique satisfies only principle one of the basic principles of shadow casting and recording unless a long PID is used. For this reason, the images created with this technique are not as accurate as those created with the parallel technique. It is, however, a satisfactory auxiliary technique that may be used when intraoral anatomy does not allow parallel film placement. When reading films exposed using the bisecting-angle technique, the practitioner must take into account the image distortion which occurs.

III. THE BISECTING-ANGLE TECHNIQUE USING FILM HOLDERS/AIMING DEVICES

Film holding with the bisecting-angle technique was originally achieved with the patient's finger. Since this method often causes film movement or bending, it is recommended that a film holder be used.

A. The Stabe Film Holder

The Stabe film holder may be used for both anterior and posterior views:

❏ For anterior views, size 0 or 1 film is positioned with its longest side in a vertical position (Fig. 9-4).

❏ For posterior adult views, size 2 film is positioned with its longest side in a horizontal position (see Fig. 9-4).

❏ The film and holder are placed behind the teeth to be examined with the film touching the lingual occlusal or incisal edge of the teeth. The patient then closes to hold the film in place (Fig. 9-5).

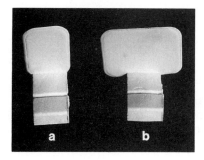

Figure 9-4. Film position in the Stabe film holder for anterior (a) and posterior (b) views. (Courtesy of Rinn Corporation, Elgin, Illinois.)

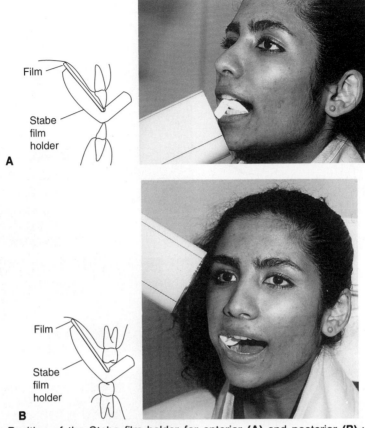

Figure 9-5. Position of the Stabe film holder for anterior **(A)** and posterior **(B)** views. (Courtesy of Rinn Corporation, Elgin, Illinois.)

❐ The vertical radiation is directed perpendicular to the imaginary line which bisects the angle formed by the tooth and film.

❐ The horizontal angulation is directed through the interproximal spaces and perpendicular to the imaginary line which extends from mesial to distal aspects of the teeth to be examined.

B. The Rinn BAI (Bisecting-Angle Instrument)

This instrument may be used with a rectangular PID or with rectangular collimating devices that attach to the aiming ring. Three instruments are needed for full-mouth periapicals:

❐ The anterior instrument holds size 0 or 1 film in a vertical position.

❐ Two posterior instruments, one for the upper right and lower left and one for the upper left and lower right, hold size 2 film in a horizontal position.

❐ Place the instrument behind the teeth to be examined. The patient should bite on the thickest part of the bite block. This will position the film against the incisal or occlusal edge of the teeth (Fig. 9-6).

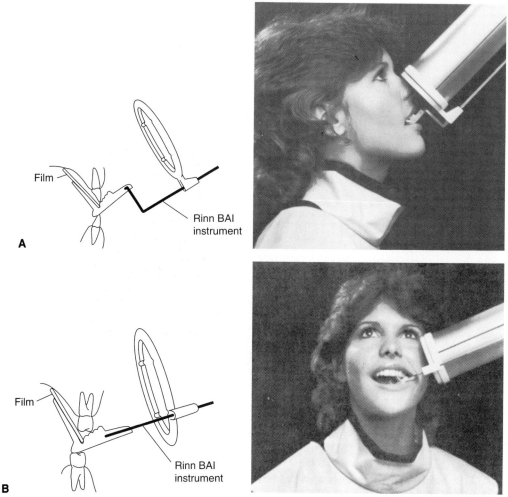

Figure 9-6. Position of the Rinn BAI film holder for anterior **(A)** and posterior **(B)** views. (Courtesy of Rinn Corporation, Elgin, Illinois.)

☐ If a round PID is used, it is positioned so that all points on its edge are equidistant from the aiming ring (see Fig. 8-7).

☐ If a rectangular PID is used, it must be turned so that its longest sides are vertical for anterior views and horizontal for posterior views. The corners of the PID must be equidistant from the notches on the aiming ring (see Fig. 8-8).

IV. FILM POSITION AND RADIATION BEAM DIRECTION FOR FULL-MOUTH PERIAPICALS USING THE BISECTING-ANGLE TECHNIQUE

The views shown in Figs. 9-7 through 9-14 are exposed on the right and left sides for a total of 16 periapical views. The number of films and film sizes in the full-mouth survey will vary with the dentist's training and preference. Views of all tooth-bearing areas must be exposed.

Text continued on page 163

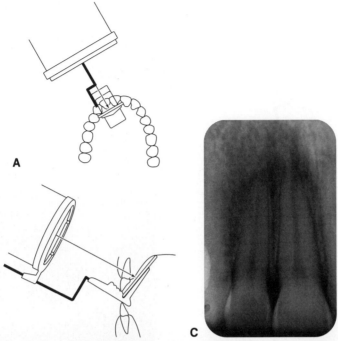

Figure 9-7. Film placement and radiation beam direction **(A, B)** for the maxillary central lateral view **(C)**. (Courtesy of Rinn Corporation, Elgin, Illinois.)

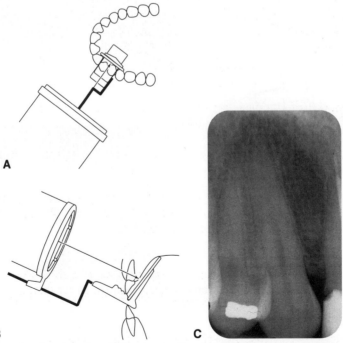

Figure 9-8. Film placement and radiation beam direction **(A, B)** for the maxillary canine view **(C)**. (Courtesy of Rinn Corporation, Elgin, Illinois.)

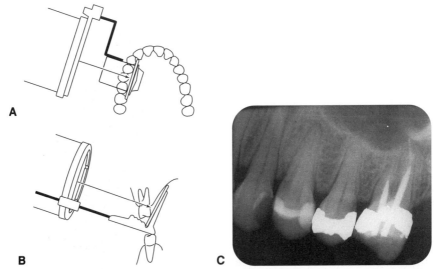

Figure 9-9. Film placement and radiation beam direction **(A, B)** for the maxillary premolar view **(C)**. (Courtesy of Rinn Corporation, Elgin, Illinois.)

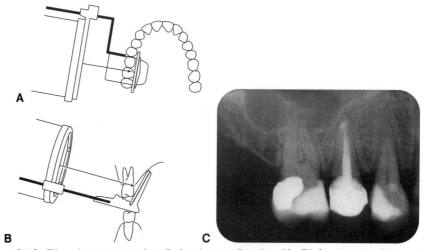

Figure 9-10. Film placement and radiation beam direction **(A, B)** for the maxillary molar view **(C)**. (Courtesy of Rinn Corporation, Elgin, Illinois.)

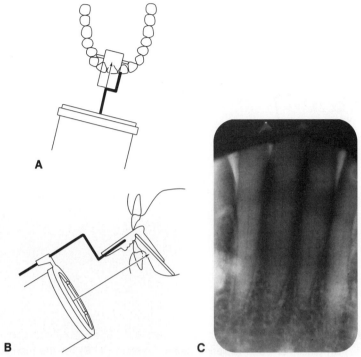

Figure 9-11. Film placement and radiation beam direction **(A, B)** for the mandibular central lateral view **(C)**. (Courtesy of Rinn Corporation, Elgin, Illinois.)

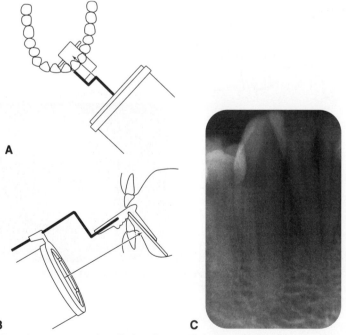

Figure 9-12. Film placement and radiation beam direction **(A, B)** for the mandibular canine view **(C)**. (Courtesy of Rinn Corporation, Elgin, Illinois.)

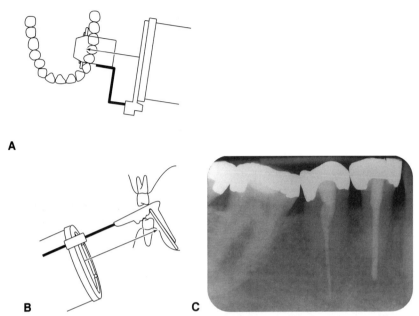

Figure 9-13. Film placement and radiation beam direction **(A, B)** for the mandibular premolar view **(C)**. (Courtesy of Rinn Corporation, Elgin, Illinois.)

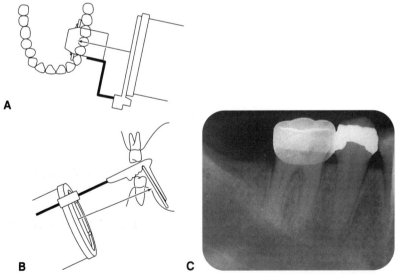

Figure 9-14. Film placement and radiation beam direction **(A, B)** for the mandibular molar view **(C)**. (Courtesy of Rinn Corporation, Elgin, Illinois.)

REVIEW EXERCISES

1. List the basic principles of the bisecting-angle technique.

2. List the basic principles of shadow casting and recording.

3. Compare the basic principles of the bisecting-angle technique and the parallel technique with those of shadow casting and recording.

4. Why is the parallel technique preferred?

5. Define the following term:

   Bisector

LEARNING ACTIVITIES

Learning Activity 9-1: Comparison of Parallel and Bisecting-Angle Techniques

Equipment:

   2 size 0 or 1 films and 2 size 2 films
   Rin XCP and BAI instruments
   DXTTR trainer

Film mounts

Periodontal probe

Location:

X-ray operatory and darkroom

Activity:

1. Expose maxillary right molar and central lateral views using the bisecting-angle technique with the Rinn BAI. Label them B.

2. Expose the same views using the parallel technique with the Rinn XCP instrument. Label them P.

3. Process the films. (Make sure that the films are correctly identified.)

4. Label and mount the films, placing the molar views side by side and the central lateral views side by side.

Questions:

1. Look at the radiographs. How do those exposed with the bisecting-angle technique differ in appearance from those taken with the parallel technique? Describe.

2. Using the periodontal probe, measure the following on the first molars and central incisors in each film:

	Parallel	Bisecting Angle
Length		
From apex of longest root to most coronal point	_____	_____
From CEJ to most coronal point	_____	_____
From CEJ to most apical point	_____	_____
Crown width from mesial to distal	_____	_____
Width		
Root width at widest point	_____	_____
Crown width at contact	_____	_____
Bone level from CEJ to crest	_____	_____

3. Explain your results.

4. Where on the tooth are the differences between the numbers the greatest? Why?

Learning Activity 9-2: Effects of Angulation and Film Positioning Changes

Equipment:

6 size 2 films

Assembled Rinn BAI film holder

Stabe film holder

Round open-ended PID (if available)

DXTTR trainer

Film mounts

Location:

X-ray operatory and darkroom

Activity:

Six exposures will be made of the maxillary premolar view (left or right) altering the vertical and horizontal angulation as well as film placement. When processed, these films will demonstrate the effect of angulation and film placement errors on films exposed with the bisecting-angle technique.

Exposure 1:
1. Place a size 2 film in the BAI bite block, and position it for the maxillary premolar view:

   behind the premolars

   thickest part of the bite block against the premolars
2. Align the PID so that all points on it are equidistant from the aiming ring. Note the vertical angulation on the side of the tube head.
3. Expose the film. Label it Exposure 1.

Exposure 2:
1. Place the film exactly as for Exposure 1.
2. Keeping the top of the PID against the top of the aiming ring, increase the vertical angulation by 10 degrees.
3. Expose the film. Label it BV+.

Exposure 3:
1. Place the film exactly as for Exposure 1.

2. Keeping the PID against the bottom of the aiming ring, decrease the vertical angulation by 10 degrees.

3. Expose the film. Label it BV−.

Exposure 4:

1. Place the film exactly as for Exposure 1.

2. Align the PID so that its right side touches the right side of the aiming ring. The left side of the PID should be 1 in away from the left side of the aiming ring.

3. Expose the film. Label it BHR.

Exposure 5:

1. Place the film exactly as for Exposure 1.

2. Align the PID so that its left side touches the left side of the aiming ring. The right side should be 1 in away from the right side of the aiming ring.

3. Expose the film. Label it BHL.

Exposure 6:

1. Using the Stabe film holder, make a larger angle between the tooth and film than in Exposure 1.

2. Direct the radiation perpendicular to the bisector of the angle and through the interproximal spaces.

3. Expose the film. Label it BFA.

Process, mount, and label the films in the order they were taken.

Questions:

1. Compare the x-ray images in films 1, BV+, and BV−. How does the image change? Why?

2. Compare the x-ray images in films 1, BHR, and BHL. How does the image change? Why?

3. Compare the x-ray images in films, 1, BV, and BH. How does the image change? Why?

4. Compare the films PV+ and PV− from Learning Activity 8-1 with the films BV+ and BV− in this activity. Do vertical angulation errors with the bisecting-angle technique differ in appearance from those with the parallel technique? Why?

5. Compare the films PHR and PHL from Learning Activity 8-1 with films BHR and BHL in this activity. Do horizontal angulation errors with the parallel technique differ in appearance from those with the bisecting-angle technique? Why?

Learning Activity 9-3: The Rinn BAI

Equipment:

>8 size 0 or 1 films, 8 size 2 films
>Rinn BAI setup for full-mouth x rays
>DXTTR trainer
>Full-mouth survey mounts

Location:

X-ray operatory and darkroom

Activity:

1. Expose all periapical views contained in an adult full-mouth survey using the bisecting-angle technique.
2. Process and mount the films.

Evaluation:

1. Examine the films for the following errors:
   Incorrect vertical angulation (V+ or V−)
   Incorrect horizontal angulation (H)
   Incorrect packet placement (P)
     Is there increased distortion due to improper film placement?
     Do the correct teeth appear in each film?
   Cone cut (C)
2. List each film that contains an error, and state the cause of the error and its correction. Circle any films that are diagnostically unacceptable and should be retaken.

Film	Error	Cause	Correction

Learning Activity 9-4: The Stabe Film Holder

Equipment:

A round open-ended PID
8 size 0 or 1 films, 8 size 2 films
Stabe film holder
DXTTR trainer
Full-mouth survey mounts

Location:

X-ray operatory and darkroom

Activity:

1. Expose all periapical views contained in an adult full-mouth survey using the bisecting-angle technique.
2. Process and mount the films.

Evaluation:

1. Examine the films for the following errors:

   Incorrect vertical angulation (V+ or V−)

   Incorrect horizontal angulation (H)

   Incorrect packet placement (P)
      Is there increased distortion due to improper film placement?
      Do the correct teeth appear in each film?

   Cone cut (C)

2. List each film that contains an error, and state the cause of the error and its correction. Circle any films that are diagnostically unacceptable and should be retaken.

Film	Error	Cause	Correction

BIBLIOGRAPHY

Frommer, Herbert H. *Radiology for Dental Auxiliaries,* 5th ed. St. Louis, Mosby–Year Book, 1992.

Goaz, Paul G., and White, Stuart C. *Oral Radiography: Principles and Interpretation.* St. Louis, C.V. Mosby, 1989.

Rinn Corporation. *Intraoral Radiography with Rinn XCP/BAI Instruments.* Elgin, Ill., Rinn Corp., 1989.

The Interproximal/Bitewing Examination

After completing this chapter the student will be able to

1. Describe the purpose of posterior, anterior, and vertical bitewing radiographs.
2. Use patient selection criteria in determining the need for bitewing radiographs.
3. Identify the number and size of films required for adequate assessment of each patient.
4. Describe and demonstrate correct bitewing technique for molar, premolar, and vertical bitewing views using

   Film tabs

   Film loops

   The Rinn instrument
5. Identify and state the cause of the following errors seen in bitewing radiographs:

   Overlapping

   Cone cut

   Sloped occlusal plane
6. Define the following term:

   Bitewing

I. PURPOSE OF BITEWINGS

Bitewing radiographs depict the crown and some of the root and surrounding bone of opposing maxillary and mandibular teeth on one film. They are used to examine the proximal surfaces of teeth for carious lesions and to evaluate the interproximal bone (Fig. 10-1). Bitewing exposures may be made of both anterior and posterior teeth.

Figure 10-1. Bitewing radiographs depict the crown and some of the root and surrounding bone of opposing maxillary and mandibular teeth on one film.

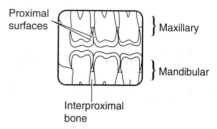

Bitewings are included in the full-mouth survey. They are also exposed during routine dental examinations at intervals determined by the patient's age, dental disease activity, and medical/dental histories (see Table 1-6).

Most bitewing examinations include premolar and molar views and may include anterior views. In a standard bitewing survey, bitewing films are used with the longest edge extending from mesial to distal aspects of the teeth (horizontal) (Fig. 10-2). If there is extensive bone loss, vertical bitewing exposures may be made. For these, the longest edge of the film extends from maxillary to mandibular (vertical) (see Fig. 10-2).

II. EQUIPMENT

A. Number and Size of Films

Unlike periapical exposures, it is not always necessary to expose bitewings in edentulous areas. Each patient must be examined to determine the size and number of films required for an adequate bitewing survey. The following guidelines may be followed for a standard (horizontal) bitewing survey:

❐ Adults with a complete dentition (may or may not include third molars) and older children with second molars will require four size 2 films for premolar and molar views on the right and left side.

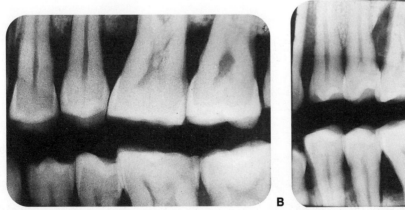

A   **B**

Figure 10-2. Vertical and horizontal bitewings. **(A)** This horizontal bitewing was exposed with the longest edge extending from mesial to distal aspects of the teeth (horizontal). **(B)** A vertical bitewing of the same area was exposed with the longest edge of the film extending from maxillary to mandibular (vertical). Because more of the root and surrounding bone can be observed in vertical bitewings, they may be used for patients with advanced bone loss.

❏ Adults with fewer teeth may require fewer films.

❏ Children with only the primary dentition will require no bitewings if the contacts are open. Two size 0 films of the right and left deciduous molars will be needed if the contacts are closed.

❏ Children with a transitional dentition (deciduous molars and first permanent molars) will require two size 0 or 1 films or one size 2 film depending on the size of the child.

❏ Size 3 film is not recommended because it is too narrow to adequately demonstrate interproximal bone levels. In addition, it is impossible to demonstrate the proximal surfaces from canine to second or third molar on one film without overlap occurring. This is so because the interproximal spaces are at different angles and it is therefore impossible to direct the radiation through all of them in one exposure.

B. Film Tabs, Holders, and Aiming Devices

In order to hold the film in its proper position, various methods are used:

❏ *Film tabs* are rectangular pieces of cardboard that attach to the middle of the film, providing a surface on which the patient bites to hold the film in place. Size 0, 1, and 2 film may be purchased with tabs in place, or adhesive tabs are available which may be attached to the film (Fig. 10-3).

❏ *Cardboard loops with tabs* are available that slip over size 0, 1, and 2 film, providing a biting tab (see Fig 10-3).

❏ The *Rinn XCP* and *BAI instruments* provide size 0, 1, and 2 vertical and horizontal bitewing holders. The Rinn instruments are recommended because they assist the operator in the proper alignment of the

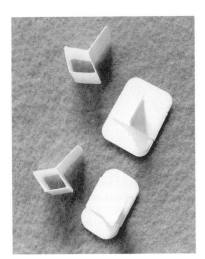

Figure 10-3. Film tabs provide a biting surface to hold the film in place.

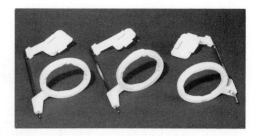

Figure 10-4. The Rinn bitewing instruments are available to hold size 0, 1, and 2 films for horizontal and vertical bitewings. (Courtesy of Rinn Corporation, Elgin, Illinois.)

film and radiation beam and may be used with rectangular collimating devices (Fig. 10-4).

Film placement is especially important with the Rinn instruments because of the relationship between film placement and radiation beam direction; if the film is placed incorrectly, the direction of the radiation beam will be incorrect.

III. TECHNIQUE

Whether tabs, loops, or the Rinn instruments are used, the same principles of film placement and radition beam direction apply.

Because bitewing radiographs are used to demonstrate the interproximal areas, correct horizontal angulation is critical. The radiation must be directed through the interproximal spaces.

Acceptable bitewings can be produced with the patient in an upright or supine position. However, it is easier to visualize the relationship between the teeth, radiation beam, and film if the patient is in an upright position with the occlusal plane parallel to the floor.

A. Adult Premolar Bitewing

This view should demonstrate the proximal spaces and interproximal bone levels from the distal of the canine to the mesial surface of the first molar (Fig. 10-5A).

Film Placement

❑ Place the film behind the mandibular premolars with its mesial edge at the middle of the mandibular canine.

❑ Position the film perpendicular to the proximal spaces of the canine, premolars, and first molar (mesial).

❑ The film should be parallel to a line drawn on the occlusal surface from the mesial side of the canine to the mesial side of the first molar.

❑ Instruct the patient to slowly close his or her mouth while ensuring that the upper edge does not impinge on the palate.

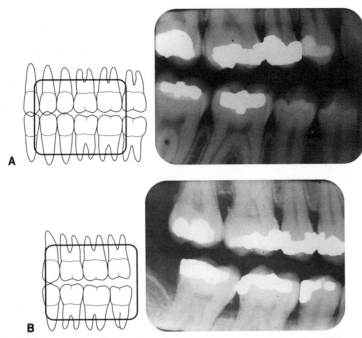

Figure 10-5. Adult premolar **(A)** and molar **(B)** bitewing radiographs. The premolar view should demonstrate the proximal spaces and interproximal bone levels from the distal side of the canines to the mesial surface of the first molar. The molar view should demonstrate the proximal surfaces and interproximal bone levels from the distal side of the second premolar to the distal side of the last erupted molar.

Radiation Beam Direction

❏ **Film tabs or loops (Fig. 10-6):**

- Center the premolars within the PID, and direct the horizontal angulation perpendicular to the end of the tab. (If the tab has been placed on the middle of the film, center it within the PID.)

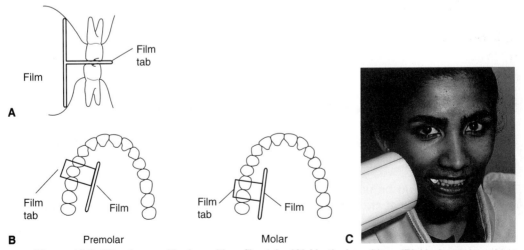

Figure 10-6. Bitewing positioning with a film tab. **(A)** Vertical position. **(B)** Horizontal position. **(C)** Patient position.

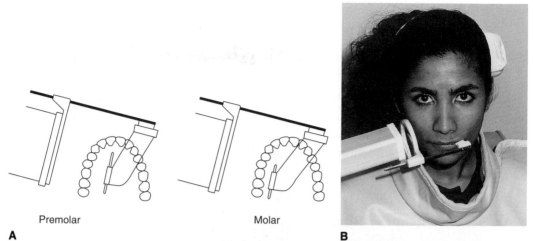

Premolar   Molar

A   **B**

Figure 10-7. Bitewing positioning with the Rinn XCP instrument. **(A)** Premolar and molar positions. **(B)** Patient position. (Courtesy of Rinn Corporation, Elgin, Illinois.)

- The vertical angulation will be at +5 to +10 if the patient's occlusal plane is parallel to the floor.

❑ **Rinn instruments (Fig. 10-7):**

- Align the PID with the aiming ring, making sure that all points on the end of the PID are equidistant from the same points on the aiming ring. If a rectangular PID is used, align the corners of the PID with the notches on the aiming ring, as with the parallel and bisecting-angle techniques.

B. Adult Molar Bitewing

This view should demonstrate the proximal surfaces and interproximal bone levels from the distal of the second premolar to the distal of the last erupted molar (see Fig. 10-5B).

Film Placement

❑ Place the film behind the mandibular molars so that the posterior edge will include the distal side of the last erupted molar in either arch.

❑ Position the film perpendicular to the proximal spaces of the molars.

❑ The film should be parallel to a line drawn on the occlusal surface from the mesial side of the first molar to the distal side of the last erupted molar.

❑ Instruct the patient to slowly close his or her mouth while ensuring that the upper part of the film does not impinge on the palate.

Radiation Beam Direction

Follow the same procedures as for the premolar bitewing.

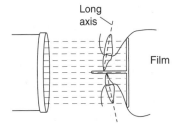

Figure 10-8. Projection geometry/anterior bitewings. The long axes of the maxillary and mandibular anterior teeth are angled differently. The film is parallel to neither, and the radiation is directed perpendicular to the film but not the teeth.

C. Pedodontic Bitewing Radiographs

❏ Follow Guidelines for Patient Selection and preceding recommendations for number and size of films.

❏ Use film tabs or Rinn instruments.

❏ Follow the same principles of technique used for adult bitewings.

D. Vertical Bitewings

❏ *Anterior vertical bitewings* are used to evaluate proximal surfaces and interproximal bone level of anterior teeth. They are taken as indicated by the patient's oral conditions and not as part of a routine examination.

❏ Anterior bitewings are less effective than posterior bitewings because of image-projection geometry. The long axes of the maxillary and mandibular anterior teeth are usually angled very differently, the film is parallel to neither, and the radiation is directed perpendicular to the film but not the teeth (Fig. 10-8).

❏ *Posterior vertical bitewings* are exposed when advanced bone loss is present which would not be demonstrated by traditional bitewing surveys.

❏ *Film size* is determined by the area to be examined. Usually size 0 or 1 film is used for anterior views and size 2 for posterior views. The Rinn instruments provide vertical bitewing holders for size 0, 1, and 2 film (Fig. 10-9).

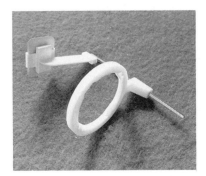

Figure 10-9. Rinn vertical bitewing holder. (Courtesy of Rinn Corporation, Elgin, Illinois.)

❏ The principles of film positioning and radiation beam direction are the same as those for traditional bitewing surveys.

E. Common Errors Seen in Bitewing Radiographs

❏ *Overlapping* is the superimposition of the mesial and distal surfaces of adjacent teeth caused by incorrect horizontal angulation (see Fig. 7-7B). Failure to place the film parallel to a line drawn on the occlusal surface through the proximal surfaces may result in overlapping if the film tab is used to align the radiation or if the Rinn instrument is used.

❏ *Cone cut* is a clear area on the film caused by failure to center the film within the PID. The edge of the image is rounded or straight depending on whether a round or rectangular PID is used. The part of the film that is not within the radiation beam is clear (see Fig. 8-2).

❏ A *sloped occlusal plane* occurs when the film strikes the sides of the palate as the patient closes his or her mouth. The occlusal plane slopes diagonally across the film instead of appearing straight across the middle of the film as it should.

❏ *Vertical angulation errors* are seen less often in bitewing radiographs. However, if too much positive vertical angulation is used, more of the maxillary arch will be projected onto the film and less of the mandibular arch will be observed. The reverse is true if too much negative vertical angulation is used.

❏ *Film placement errors* are seen most frequently in a failure to place the film far enough anteriorly, thereby missing the adjacent proximal surfaces of the canine and first premolar.

REVIEW EXERCISES

1. Describe the purpose of posterior, anterior, and vertical bitewing radiographs.

2. Describe the number and size of radiographs, if any, that should be exposed during the first dental visit of a 4-year-old patient with open contacts and no evidence of dental disease. Why?

3. Describe the number and size of radiographs, if any, that should be exposed on a 45-year-old patient with a complete dentition and clinical

findings of occlusal carious lesions on teeth 6, 14, 18, and 32, generalized bleeding on probing, and generalized pocket depths of 3 to 4 mm.
(The patient's last dental visit was 2 years ago when a full-mouth survey was taken.) Why? *4 BWX) selected PA*

4. Describe the correct bitewing technique for molar, premolar, and bitewing views using

   film tabs

   film loops

   the Rinn instrument

5. Identify and state the cause of the following errors seen in bitewing
   radiographs:

   The proximal surfaces are superimposed. *incorrect horizontal angulation*

   There is a curved clear area on the anterior portion of the film. *Cone cut Failure to center film to x* *film strikes palate*

   The occlusal plane is on an angle across the film. *as pt closes mouth tilting film.*

6. Define the following term:

   Bitewing

LEARNING ACTIVITIES

Learning Activity 10-1: Effects of Angulation Changes

Equipment:

   Rinn XCP bitewing instrument for size 2 film
   DXTTR trainer
   Round, open-ended PID
   Rectangular PID
   Radiograph view box

Location:

X-ray operatory and darkroom

Activity:

Exposure 1:

1. Using the Rinn bitewing instrument with size 2 film, place the film in the DXTTR mannequin for a premolar bitewing view:

    behind the premolars with the anterior edge at the middle of the canine.

    perpendicular to the proximal spaces of the premolars, canine, and first molar.

2. Align the PID so that all points on it are equidistant from the aiming ring. Note the degree of vertical angulation on the number scale.

3. Expose the film. Label it Exposure 1.

Exposure 2:

1. Place the film exactly as for Exposure 1.

2. Align the PID so that the anterior edge touches the corresponding edge of the aiming ring; the posterior edge should be approximately ½ in away from the aiming ring.

3. Adjust the vertical angulation to that used in Exposure 1.

4. Expose the film. Label it Exposure 2.

Exposure 3:

1. Place the film exactly as for Exposure 1.

2. Align the PID so that the anterior edge touches the anterior edge of the aiming ring; the posterior edge should be approximately 1 in away from the aiming ring.

3. Adjust the vertical angulation to that used in Exposure 1.

4. Expose the film. Label it Exposure 3.

Exposure 4:

1. Place the film exactly as for Exposure 1.

2. Align the PID so that the posterior edge touches the posterior edge of the aiming ring; the anterior edge should be approximately ½ in away from the aiming ring.

3. Adjust the vertical angulation to that used in Exposure 1.

4. Expose the film. Label it Exposure 4.

Exposure 5:

1. Place the film exactly as for Exposure 1.

2. Align the PID so that the posterior edge touches the posterior edge of the aiming ring; the anterior edge should be approximately 1 in away from the aiming ring.

3. Adjust the vertical angulation to that used in Exposure 1.

4. Expose the film. Label it Exposure 5.

Exposure 6:
1. Place the film exactly as for Exposure 1.
2. Align the PID so that its upper edge touches the upper edge of the aiming ring; its lower edge should be 1 in away from the lower edge of the aiming ring.
3. Adjust the horizontal angulation so that the anterior and posterior edges of the PID are equidistant from the aiming ring.
4. Expose the film. Label it Exposure 6.

Exposure 7:
1. Place the film exactly as for Exposure 1.
2. Align the PID so that its lower edge touches the lower edge of the aiming ring; its upper edge should be 1 in away from the upper edge of the aiming ring.
3. Adjust the horizontal angulation so that the anterior and posterior edges are equidistant from the aiming ring.
4. Expose the film. Label it Exposure 7.

Exposure 8:
1. Place the film exactly as for Exposure 1.
2. Align the PID so that all points on it are equidistant from the aiming ring. Now move it distally 1 in.
3. Expose the film. Label it Exposure 8.

Exposure 9:
1. Attach the rectangular PID.
2. Place the film exactly as for Exposure 1.
3. Align the PID so that its four corners are equidistant from the notches on the aiming ring. Now move it distally 1 in.
4. Expose the film. Label it Exposure 9.

Process the films, being sure to label each with its correct number. Mount the films in the order in which they were taken.

Questions:

1. Compare the appearance of films 1 to 5.

   What teeth appear in each film?

   If the film placement is the same for each exposure, why do different teeth appear in the films?

   How does each film differ?

   What is the technical error caused by incorrect horizontal angulation?

2. Compare the appearance of films 1, 6, and 7.

   How do the films differ?

   Why?

3. Compare the appearance of films 1, 8, and 9.

   How do they differ?

   Why?

   What is this technical error called? *Cone cut*

Learning Activity 10-2: Comparison of Horizontal and Vertical Bitewings

Equipment:

Rinn XCP horizontal bitewing instrument for size 2 film

Rinn XCP vertical bitewing instrument for size 2 film

Rinn XCP vertical bitewing instrument for size 0 or 1 film

DXTTR trainer

View box

Location:

X-ray operatory and darkroom

Activity:

1. Expose a premolar and molar bitewing using the horizontal bitewing instrument.
2. Expose vertical bitewings of the same areas using the vertical bitewing instruments for both size 2 and 0/1 film.
3. Process and mount the films.

Question:

Compare the films. Assess

adequacy of visibility of proximal surfaces for each.

adequacy of visibility of bone level for each.

the advantages and disadvantages of each.

Learning Activity 10-3: The Rinn XCP Instrument

Equipment:

Rinn XCP instrument for size 2 film
DXTTR trainer

Location:

X-ray operatory and darkroom

Activity:

1. Expose a complete adult bitewing survey (right and left pre-molar and molar views).
2. Process and mount the films.

Questions:

1. Evaluate the films for technical errors. State the error and describe its cause and correction.

Film	Error	Cause	Correction

2. Should any films be retaken? Why?

BIBLIOGRAPHY

Frommer, Herbert H. *Radiology for Dental Auxiliaries,* 5th ed. St. Louis, Mosby–Year Book, 1992.

Goaz, Paul G., and White, Stuart C. *Oral Radiography: Principles and Interpretation.* St. Louis, C.V. Mosby, 1989.

Rinn Corporation. *Intraoral Radiography with Rinn XCP/BAI Instruments.* Elgin, Ill., Rinn Corp., 1989.

Auxiliary Radiographic Techniques

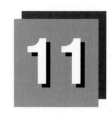

After completing this chapter the student will be able to

1. Describe the uses for occlusal radiographs.
2. Describe and demonstrate the technique for exposing topographic and cross-sectional occlusal radiographs.
3. Describe and demonstrate the following localization techniques:

   Tube shift

   Right angle
4. Describe the function of intensifying screens in extraoral radiography.
5. Describe the uses for panoramic radiographs.
6. Describe the advantages and disadvantages of panoramic radiographs.
7. Describe and demonstrate the technique for exposing panoramic radiographs.
8. Describe dual, triple, and moving-center rotation in panoramic x-ray machines.
9. Identify and state the cause of common errors in panoramic radiographs.
10. Locate the following on the panoramic radiograph:

Middle cranial fossa	External oblique line
Orbit	Angle of the mandible
Zygomatic arch	Hyoid bone
Palate	Glenoid fossa
Styloid process	Articular eminence
Septa in the maxillary sinus	Mandibular condyle
	Vertebra
Maxillary tuberosity	Coronoid process

Pterygoid plates   Mandibular canal

Maxillary sinus   Mental foramen

Earlobe

11. Describe the use and technique for the following extraoral projections:

Lateral oblique   Posteroanterior

Lateral skull   Transcranial TMJ

Cephalometric

12. Define the following terms:

Fluorescent   Phosphor

Focal trough   Rotation center

Frankfort plane   Scanography

Midsaggital plane   Tomography

I. OCCLUSAL RADIOGRAPHS

Occlusal radiographs are used to view large areas of the maxilla or mandible that cannot be demonstrated in periapical radiographs. They may be used alone or in conjunction with bitewing, periapical, or panoramic radiographs to localize objects, identify pathologic conditions, and assess growth and development of the teeth and jaws. Size 4 film is usually used for adult exposures, while size 2 film may be used for occlusal projections on small children (Fig. 11-1). There are two types of occlusal projections.

A. Topographic Occlusal Radiographs

Topographic occlusal radiographs have the appearance of a large periapical film (Fig. 11-2). This type of occlusal projection is used when periapical exposures demonstrate insufficient area, when periapical film placement is impossible, or to reduce radiation exposure when assessing edentulous areas or the deciduous dentition.

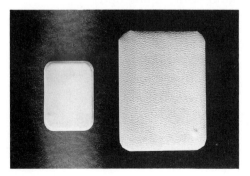

Figure 11-1. Occlusal film (sizes 4 and 2). Size 4 film is usually used for adult exposures, while size 2 film may be used for occlusal projections on small children.

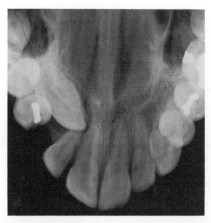

Figure 11-2. Topographic occlusal projection. This projection has the appearance of a large periapical film. It is used to demonstrate larger areas than can be viewed on periapical film or to reduce the number of exposures required to view edentulous areas or the deciduous dentition. (From Miles DA, et al: *Radiographic Imaging for Dental Auxiliaries,* 2d ed. Philadelphia, W.B. Saunders Company, 1993. P. 140.)

❐ **Patient position.** The patient should be in an upright position with the occlusal plane parallel to the floor (Fig. 11-3).

❐ **Film placement.** The film is placed across the occlusal surfaces of the teeth with the area to be examined centered in the film. The plain side of the film should face the area to be examined and the radiation source (see Fig. 11-3).

❐ **PID.** Because of the large size of occlusal film, a round, open-ended PID must be used. It may be long, intermediate, or short.

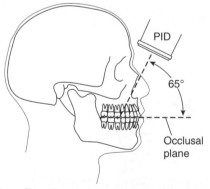

Figure 11-3. Patient position, film placement, and radiation beam direction for topographic occlusal views. The patient should be in an upright position with the occlusal plane parallel to the floor. The film is placed across the occlusal surfaces with the area to be examined centered in the film. The vertical angulation will vary from 45 to 75 degrees depending on the area being examined.

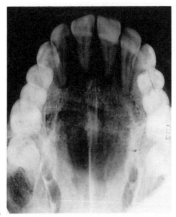
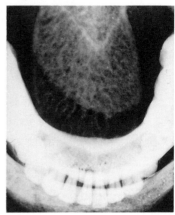

A   **B**

Figure 11-4. Cross-sectional occlusal projections of the maxilla **(A)** and mandible **(B)**. In this projection, the teeth have a round or elliptical appearance. A cross-sectional occlusal projection may be used to locate teeth, objects, or pathology, to view large pathologic lesions, or to assess changes in the size and shape of the arches or tori.

- ❏ **Radiation beam direction.** The bisecting-angle technique is used. Angulation will vary from 45 to 75 degrees depending on the area to be examined (see Fig. 11-3).

B. Cross-Sectional Occlusal Radiographs

A cross section of the arch is demonstrated by a *cross-sectional occlusal radiograph* (Fig. 11-4). Because of the direction of the radiation beam (below), the tooth structure is superimposed on itself from apex to crown, giving the teeth a round or elliptical appearance. A cross-sectional occlusal projection may be used to locate teeth, objects, or pathology, to view large pathologic lesions, or to assess changes in the size and shape of the arches or tori.

- ❏ **Patient position.** For maxillary exposures, the patient should be in an upright position with the occlusal plane parallel to the floor (Fig. 11-5). For mandibular exposures, the patient's head should be tilted back, or the patient may be in a supine position (see Fig. 11-5).

- ❏ **Film placement.** The film is placed across the occlusal surfaces of the teeth with the area to be examined centered in the film. The plain side of the film should face the area to be examined and the radiation source (see Fig 11-5).

- ❏ **PID.** Because of the large size of occlusal film, a round, open-ended PID must be used. It may be long, intermediate, or short.

- ❏ **Radiation beam direction.** The radiation is directed perpendicular to the film (see Fig. 11-5).

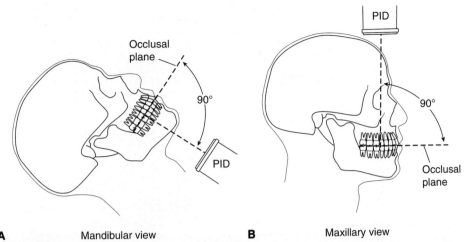

A   Mandibular view   **B**   Maxillary view

Figure 11-5. Patient position, film placement, and radiation beam direction for cross-sectional occlusal views. For mandibular exposures **(A)**, the patient's head should be tilted back or the patient may be in a supine position. For maxillary exposures **(B)**, the patient should be in an upright position with the occlusal plane parallel to the floor. The film is placed across the occlusal surfaces. The vertical angulation is directed perpendicular to the film.

II. LOCALIZATION TECHNIQUES

Dental radiographs are two-dimensional representations of three-dimensional objects. The superoinferior and anteroposterior relationships of objects can be observed in periapical films, but the buccal-lingual relationship cannot. Cross-sectional occlusal films demonstrate anteroposterior and buccal-lingual relationships but not the superoinferior relationships. When it is necessary to identify the location of a foreign object, impacted teeth, or other conditions, two methods are used.

A. The Right-Angle Technique

Two films are exposed at right angles to each other to identify the location of an object. As previously described, periapical radiographs demonstrate superoinferior and anteroposterior positions of objects. Cross-sectional occlusal radiographs demonstrate the anteroposterior and buccal-lingual positions. By exposing these two radiographic views in an area, all three dimensions of the area will be demonstrated, and the location of objects can be identified (Fig. 11-6).

B. The Tube-Shift Technique

The principle of this technique is also called the *buccal object rule* or *Clark's rule,* after C. A. Clark, who first described it in 1910.

Two periapical radiographs are exposed in an area. The horizontal angulation is altered by approximately 20 degrees mesially or distally in the second exposure. Objects closer to the buccal surface will move in the opposite direction from the tube head movement or shift. Objects on the lingual surface will move in the same direction as the tube head movement (Fig. 11-7).

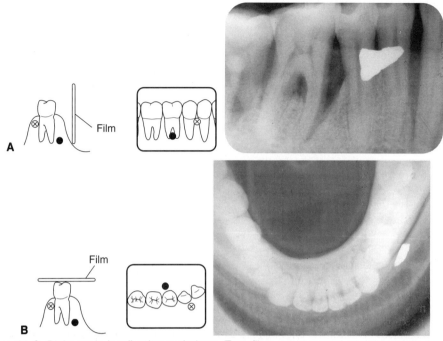

Figure 11-6. Right-angle localization technique. Two films are exposed at right angles to each other to identify the location of an object. The periapical radiograph **(A)** will demonstrate the superoinferior and anteroposterior positions of objects. A cross-sectional occlusal radiograph **(B)** will demonstrate the anteroposterior and buccal-lingual positions. These two radiographic views will demonstrate all three dimensions of an area, and the location of objects can be identified.

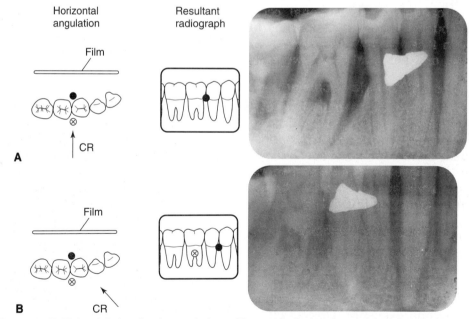

Figure 11-7. Tube-shift localization technique. Two periapical radiographs are exposed in an area. One **(A)** is exposed with correct horizontal angulation, and the second **(B)** is exposed altering the horizontal angulation by approximately 20 degrees mesially. The object moved in the opposite direction (distal) from the tube shift and therefore is located on the buccal aspect.

For example, if the horizontal angulation is changed by moving the tube head to the mesial, objects on the lingual surface will move mesially, while those on the buccal surface will move distally. This can be remembered with the acronym *SLOB: same lingual, opposite buccal.*

III. EXTRAORAL PROJECTIONS

The majority of dental radiographs are exposed intraorally; however, there is occasionally a need to observe structures that cannot be demonstrated in intraoral radiographs. Extraoral projections are used for this purpose.

A. Equipment

❐ **The x-ray machine.** Extraoral films are exposed using a standard dental x-ray unit. For most projections, a TFD of 36 in is needed with a round, open-ended PID to obtain a beam sufficiently large to expose the anatomic structures and film. KVp, mA, and exposure times vary with the projection.

❐ **The film cassette.** Either flexible or rigid, the film cassette holds the extraoral film and protects it from light exposure yet allows the passage of x rays (Fig. 11-8). Cassettes come in various sizes corresponding to the sizes of extraoral film (usually 5×7 or 8×10 in). The cassettes are marked with lead letters *L* or *R* to identify the patient's left or right side.

❐ **Intensifying screens.** As their name suggests, intensifying screens intensify the effect of radiation on the film and therefore reduce the amount of radiation required to properly expose the film. The screens are coated with a **fluorescent** material, a substance that emits light

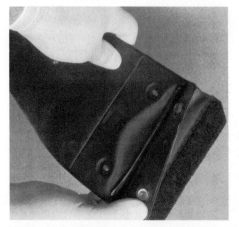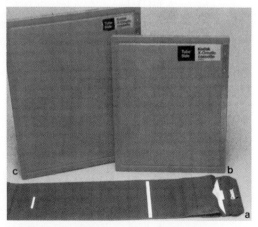

Figure 11-8. The film cassette holds the extraoral film and protects it from light exposure yet allows the passage of x rays. (a) A flexible 5- by 12-in panoramic cassette. (b) An 8- by 10-in cassette for lateral cephalometric and other extraoral views. (c) A 10- by 14-in cassette for extraoral views. (From Miles DA, et al: *Radiographic Imaging for Dental Auxiliaries,* 2d ed. Philadelphia, W.B. Saunders Company, 1993. P. 160.)

when it interacts with radiation, called a **phosphor.** The pattern of light emitted by the screen is the same as the pattern of radiation which has passed through the object. The film, sandwiched between intensifying screens, is exposed by both light and radiation. Two types of phosphors are *calcium tungstate* and *rare earth elements.*

- *Calcium tungstate* was for years the most commonly used phosphor. It produces a blue light and is slower than newer rare earth phosphors. It must be used with compatible extraoral film that is sensitive to blue light.

- *Rare earth elements* are now used as intensifying screen phosphors. They reduce patient exposure by converting x-ray energy to light four times faster than calcium tungstate. Rare earth screens must be used with film sensitive to the green light emitted when they are exposed to radiation. Rare earth screens are recommended because of the reduction in patient radiation exposure.

❏ **Cassette-holding devices.** While the film cassette may be held by the patient, holding devices minimize errors caused by patient or film movement and aid in standardizing exposure technique. Cassette holding devices may be wall-mounted or free-standing.

❏ **Grids.** The amount of scatter radiation reaching the film is reduced by grids, thereby improving image quality (Fig. 11-9). They are placed between the patient and the film and absorb any radiation that is not at right angles to the film. Grids are used routinely with medical x-ray units. They are not used routinely with dental x-ray units.

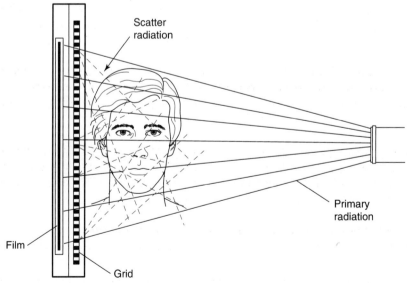

Figure 11-9. Film grid. The amount of scatter radiation reaching the film is reduced by the film grid. It is placed between the patient and the film to absorb any radiation that is not at right angles to the film.

B. Processing Extraoral Radiographs

❏ **Safelighting.** Extraoral films are more sensitive to light than are intraoral films. Safelighting which is adequate for intraoral films may ruin extraoral films. The Kodak GBX-2 safelight filter equipped with a 15-W bulb positioned 3 to 4 ft from the work surface will provide safelighting for both intra- and extraoral radiographs.

❏ **Film/cassette handling.**

• *Film.* Handle the film by its edges to avoid fingerprints. Use care if processing more than one film to avoid films touching and/or scratching.

• *Cassette.* Film cassettes which come in contact with the patient should be disinfected and/or wrapped. Care must be taken not to scratch the intensifying screen when inserting and removing the film. If the phosphor is removed by scratching, white streaks will appear on the radiograph. Damaged screens and cassettes must be discarded.

❏ **Processing.** Extraoral films are processed in the same manner as intraoral films using either manual processing and the time-temperature method or an automatic processor large enough to accommodate extraoral film.

C. Panoramic Radiographs

Panoramic radiographs (Fig. 11-10) demonstrate the entire maxilla and mandible on one film. They are used as an adjunct to full-mouth and bitewing surveys to assess these areas for pathology and anomalies and to monitor growth and development. Panoramic radiographs demonstrate generally poorer image quality than either the full-mouth or bitewing survey and should not be used as a replacement for either. They are exposed using two radiographic principles: **tomography** and **scanography.**

❏ *Tomography* demonstrates a layer of tissue on film while blurring out other layers. The **focal trough** (Fig. 11-11) is the three-dimensional area where objects must be positioned to be clearly demonstrated. Objects outside of this area will be blurred.

❏ *Scanography* produces an x-ray image by scanning an object with a narrow beam of x rays. A scatter guard protects the film from exposure to scatter radiation. The primary beam passes through an opening in the scatter guard which moves with the x-ray beam to expose the film.

❏ *Curved-layer tomography,* also known as *rotational panoramic radiography,* combines these two principles to expose panoramic radiographs:

• The x-ray film carrier and the x-ray tube head are connected and rotate simultaneously around the patient at a pivotal point called a **rotation center.**

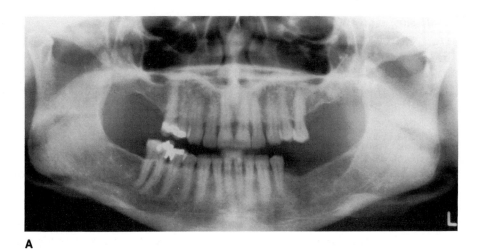

A

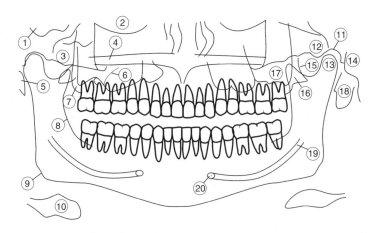

(1)	Middle cranial fossa	(11)	Glenoid fossa
(2)	Orbit	(12)	Articular eminence
(3)	Zygomatic arch	(13)	Mandibular condyle
(4)	Palate	(14)	Vertebra
(5)	Styloid process	(15)	Coronoid process
(6)	Septa in maxillary sinus	(16)	Pterygoid plates
(7)	Maxillary tuberosity	(17)	Maxillary sinus
(8)	External oblique line	(18)	Ear lobe
(9)	Angle of mandible	(19)	Mandibular canal
(10)	Hyoid bone	(20)	Mental foramen

B

Figure 11-10. Panoramic radiograph **(A)**, panoramic anatomy **(B)**. (Part *A* from Miles DA, et al: Radiographic Imaging for Dental Auxiliaries, 2d ed. Philadelphia, W.B. Saunders Company, 1993. P. 163.)

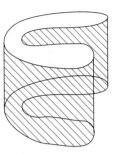

Figure 11-11. The focal trough is the three-dimensional area where objects must be positioned to be clearly demonstrated.

- The radiation emerges from the tube head as a vertical slit, passes through the patient and the vertical slit in the film carrier, and records objects located in the focal trough on the film.

- The film and tube head move at the same speed in opposite directions so that as the radiation passes through an area, the area is recorded on the film.

D. Types of Panoramic X-ray Machines

All the various panoramic x-ray machines available use intensifying screens with a film size of either 5×12 or 6×12 in. They differ mainly in the number and location of rotational centers used in exposing the radiograph, whether the focal spot is fixed or adjustable, the type and shape of the film transport mechanism, and patient positioning.

The number and location of rotational centers influence the location and size of the focal trough. The location and size of the focal trough is important to patient positioning, since only those structures positioned within the focal trough will be clearly and accurately demonstrated in the radiograph.

❏ *Double-center rotation machines*, as the name implies, have two rotational centers, one for the right and one for the left side of the jaws (Fig. 11-12A). The machine is turned off and the patient's position is shifted when the rotational center is changed. This results in an unexposed area in the center of the film. This system creates a wide focal trough (Fig. 11-13A) which has medially curving distal ends. This results in decreased sharpness in the temporomandibular joint (TMJ) area.

❏ *Triple-center rotation machines* have three centers of rotation and create an uninterrupted radiographic image of the jaws (see Fig. 11-12B). The focal trough created by this system (see Fig. 11-13B) is wide at the posterior and narrow at the anterior. The anterior teeth must be positioned very carefully to achieve optimal sharpness.

❏ *Moving-center rotation machines* (see Fig. 11-12C) rotate around a continuously moving center which is similar in shape to the arches. The size of the path may be altered to match the size of the arch being examined. An uninterrupted image of the jaws is created. The focal trough (see Fig. 11-13C) is narrow anteriorly and wide posteriorly, creating a sharp TMJ image. Careful patient positioning is required.

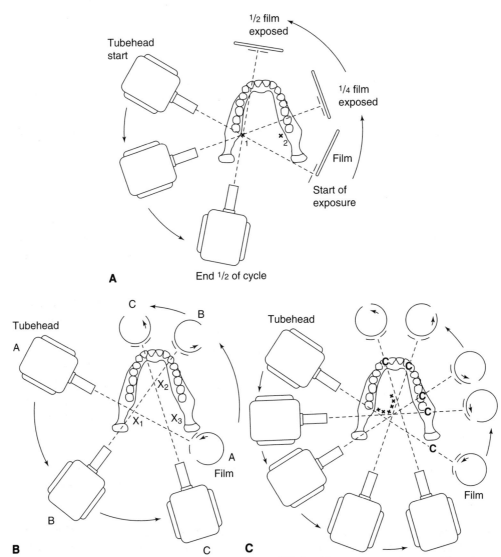

Figure 11-12. Types of panoramic x-ray machines. **(A)** Double-center rotation machines have two rotational centers, one for the right and one for the left side of the jaws. **(B)** Triple-center rotation machines have three centers of rotation and create an uninterrupted radiographic image of the jaws. **(C)** Moving-center rotation machines rotate around a continuously moving center which is similar in shape to the arches, creating an uninterrupted image of the jaws.

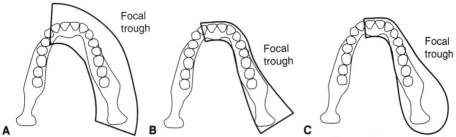

Figure 11-13. Double-, triple-, and moving-center rotation focal troughs. **(A)** The double-center rotation system creates a wide focal trough which has medially curving distal ends resulting in decreased sharpness in the TMJ area. **(B)** The focal trough created by the triple-center rotation system is wide at the posterior and narrow at the anterior. The anterior teeth must be positioned very carefully to achieve optimum sharpness. **(C)** The focal trough created by the moving-center rotation system is narrow anteriorly and wide posteriorly creating a sharp TMJ image. Careful positioning of the anterior teeth is required.

E. Exposing Panoramic Radiographs

The many panoramic x-ray machines available require slightly different procedures for patient positioning and exposure. Carefully read the manufacturer's directions before exposing radiographs. In general, the following steps should be followed:

❏ **Infection control.** Cover and/or disinfect any part of the machine that comes in contact with the patient. Sterilize any part that comes in contact with blood or saliva (see Chap. 2).

❏ **Cassette preparation.** In the darkroom, under proper safelight conditions, label the film with the patient's name and date. Carefully load it into the cassette. Be sure that it is tightly closed before it is exposed to white light. Load the cassette into the cassette holder following manufacturer's directions.

❏ **Patient preparation.** Have the patient remove jewelry, eyeglasses, and dental appliances that will interfere with the radiographic image, and explain the procedure to the patient.

❏ **Patient positioning.** Some aspects of patient position may differ from machine to machine or may change depending on the area to be radiographed. However, for all panoramic projections the **midsaggital plane** (Fig.11-14), which divides the body in half into right and left sides, must be *perpendicular* to the floor. The **Frankfort plane** (see Fig 11-14), which passes through the floor of the orbit and the external auditory meatus, must be *parallel* to the floor.

❏ *Expose the radiograph* following the manufacturer's instructions.

❏ *Process the radiograph* as you would an intraoral film.

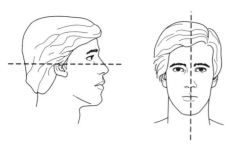

Figure 11-14. Frankfort and midsaggital planes. The Frankfort plane passes through the floor of the orbit and the external auditory meatus. The mid-saggital plane divides the body in half into right and left sides.

Frankfort plane   Mid-saggital plane

F. Common Errors in Panoramic Radiography

Most errors in panoramic radiography are caused by improper patient position. Such errors can be avoided by taking time to explain the procedure to the patient and to carefully follow the manufacturer's instructions for patient positioning. Here are some things to keep in mind:

☐ *The distance from the tube head to the object determines the location of the focal trough.*

☐ *The width of the focal trough is determined by the distance from the rotation center to the object.* The focal trough widens as the distance from the rotation center to the object increases.

☐ *The sharpness of the image decreases as the object moves from the center of the focal trough.* As objects are positioned farther from the center of the focal trough, their image becomes increasingly blurred.

☐ *Objects that are placed posterior to the center of the focal trough will appear wider in the radiograph.* If the patient is positioned too far back, the anterior teeth appear blurred and widened.

☐ *Objects positioned anterior to the center of focal trough will appear narrower in the radiograph.* If the patient is positioned too far forward, the anterior teeth will appear blurred and narrow. Increased overlapping of the premolars will be evident, and the spinal column will be superimposed on the ramus.

☐ *The Frankfort plane should be parallel to the floor.* If the patient's head is tilted up, the forehead will be too far back and the chin too far forward (Fig. 11-15). The mandibular incisors will be centered in the focal trough; however, the maxillary incisors will not and will appear blurred and widened. The palate will be superimposed on the apices of the maxillary teeth. The condyles will be close to the lateral border or off the film. The occlusal plane will appear straight across the radiograph. If the patient's head is tilted too far down, the lower incisors will be blurred and widened, and the apices of the maxillary incisors will appear much below the palate (Fig. 11-16). The middle of the occlusal plane will have an exaggerated downward curvature, and the condyles will be demonstrated more medially.

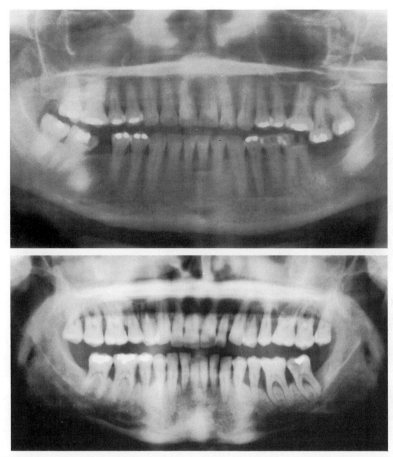

Figure 11-15. Two examples of the patient's chin being too far forward. (From Miles DA, et al: *Radiographic Imaging for Dental Auxiliaries,* 2d ed. Philadelphia, W.B. Saunders Company, 1993. P. 171.)

❑ *The midsaggital plane should be perpendicular to the floor and in the middle of the head positioner.* Areas close to the film will be smaller and exhibit increased density, while those farther away will be magnified and exhibit decreased density (Fig. 11-17).

❑ *The patient must be instructed to sit or stand still in an erect position and to hold the tongue against the palate.* Movement during exposure causes blurring of the part of the image which is being recorded at the time of movement (Fig. 11-18). Movement of the image of anatomic structures occurs as they are moved, creating unusual panoramic radiographs. If the patient does not sit or stand with the cervical spine erect, it will be curved. This will be demonstrated in the radiograph as a triangular-shaped radiopacity superimposed on the anterior teeth. Failure to hold the tongue against the palate creates an air space that will be observed in the radiograph as a radiolucent band superimposed on the apices of the maxillary anterior teeth (Fig. 11-19).

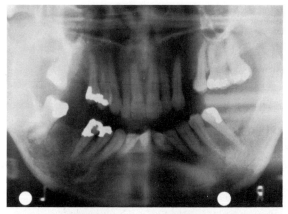

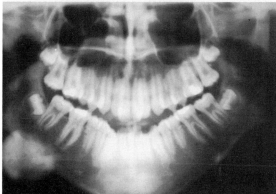

Figure 11-16. Two examples of the patient's chin being too far down. (From Miles DA, et al: *Radiographic Imaging for Dental Auxiliaries,* 2d ed. Philadelphia, W.B. Saunders Company, 1993. P. 168.)

Figure 11-17. An example in which the right side of the mandible (*RM*) is magnified because it is further away from the film than the left side. (From Miles DA, et al: *Radiographic Imaging for Dental Auxiliaries,* 2d ed. Philadelphia, W.B. Saunders Company, 1993. P. 170.)

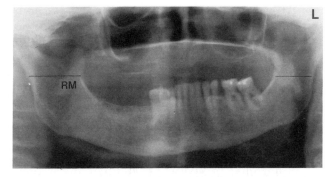

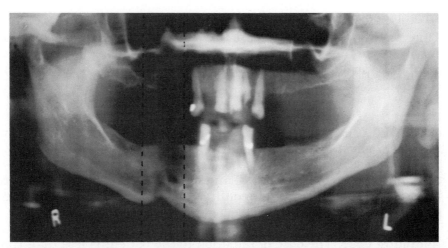

Figure 11-18. An example of the patient moving during exposure, creating a distorted band running from top to bottom. (From Miles DA, et al: *Radiographic Imaging for Dental Auxiliaries,* 2d ed. Philadelphia, W.B. Saunders Company, 1993. P. 173.)

☐ *Ensure that the film cassette does not touch the patient during exposure.* If the cassette touches the patient and slows down during the exposure, radiolucent bands will be created in the areas of overexposure. After positioning the patient, run the machine without radiation to ensure that the cassette will not touch.

☐ *Remove all dental appliances, jewelry, and chains.* Their images and their ghost may interfere with interpretation of the radiograph.

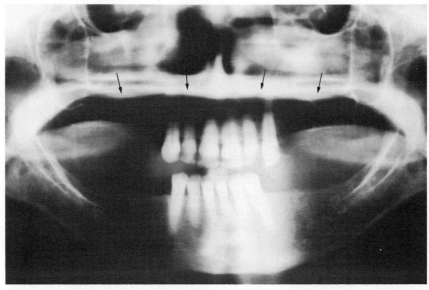

Figure 11-19. An example of the patient failing to hold tongue against the palate, creating the black area over the root apices of the maxillary teeth. (From Miles DA, et al: *Radiographic Imaging for Dental Auxiliaries,* 2d ed. Philadelphia, W.B. Saunders Company, 1993. P. 169.)

G. Advantages of Panoramic Radiography

❐ **Time saving.** The time required to expose and process a panoramic survey is far less than that required for individual periapical radiographs. Because panoramic films are not mounted, mounting time is eliminated.

❐ **Patient comfort.** Since film placement is extraoral, there is less patient discomfort, especially in the presence of a severe gag reflex, than with intraoral radiographs.

❐ **Size of area demonstrated.** Panoramic radiographs demonstrate a much larger area than a full-mouth survey. This may reveal conditions that would not be otherwise detected.

❐ **Radiation dose.** The dose of radiation to the patient is less than that of a full-mouth survey exposed with E speed film and rectangular collimation but more than a bitewing survey taken under those conditions.

H. Disadvantages of Panoramic Radiography

❐ **Image quality.** The panoramic image demonstrates uneven magnification, distortion, and poor definition. This does not interfere with its value in assessing growth and development, fractures, tumors, impacted teeth, and other pathology. However, the panoramic image is not adequate for the identification of incipient caries, interrupted lamina dura, crestal irregularities, or other conditions that require high image quality for their detection.

❐ **Overlapping.** Overlap is common, especially in the premolar area.

❐ **Superimposition.** The spinal column is commonly superimposed on areas of interest.

❐ **Ghost images.** Blurred images of the jaws called *ghost images* are repeated higher and on the opposite side of the radiograph from their actual image (Fig. 11-20). Ghost images and other artifacts may interfere with interpretation.

I. The Lateral Oblique Survey

The *lateral oblique survey* (Fig. 11-21), also known as the *lateral jaw survey,* demonstrates one side of the mandible and/or the maxilla from the distal side of the canine to the angle, ramus, condyle, and coronoid process. It is used to identify large lesions or impacted teeth, especially third molars. A standard dental x-ray unit equipped with a round, open-ended PID may be used to make the projections.

❐ **Film size.** Occlusal film may be used for small children. For adult projections, 5 × 7 or 8 × 10 in extraoral films in cassettes are used.

❐ **Cassette position.** The cassette may be placed in a cassette holder or held by the patient between the palm and the cheekbone as it rests on

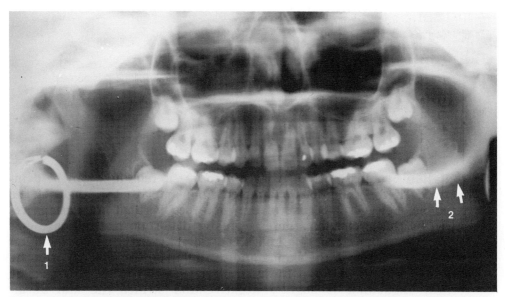

Figure 11-20. Panoramic ghost images are blurred images of the jaws repeated higher and on the opposite side of the radiograph from their actual image [in this case, an earring left on mistakenly (1) is repeated as a ghost image on the opposite side (2)]. (From Haring JI, Lind LJ: *Radiographic Interpretation for the Dental Hygienist.* Philadelphia, W.B. Saunders Company, 1993. P. 73.)

the shoulder. It is placed on the side of the face to be examined and in contact with the cheekbone and ear if the ramus is the area of interest or the cheekbone and mandible if the body of the mandible is the area of interest. It should extend at least 1 in beyond the inferior border of the mandible.

◻ **Patient position.** The patient is seated. To begin, the occlusal plane should be parallel to the floor, and the midsaggital plane should be perpendicular to the floor. The chin then should be extended forward to move the mandible away from the spine, and the head should be tilted approximately 15 degrees toward the cassette (Fig. 11-22).

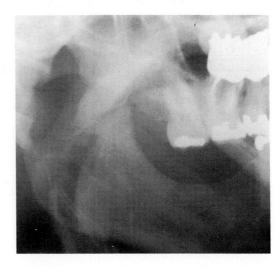

Figure 11-21. The lateral oblique survey, also known as the *lateral jaw survey,* demonstrates one side of the mandible and/or the maxilla from the distal of the canine to the angle, ramus, condyle and coronoid process. (From Miles DA, et al: *Radiographic Imaging for Dental Auxiliaries,* 2d ed. Philadelphia, W.B. Saunders Company, 1993. P. 182.)

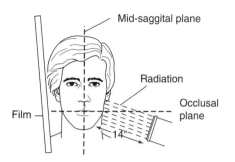

Figure 11-22. Lateral oblique positioning.

❏ **Radiation beam direction.** A large area of the mandible can be demonstrated if the radiation is directed from beneath the angle of the mandible; however, because of the increased vertical angulations required by this projection, there is greater distortion of the image (see Fig. 11-22). A more accurate image is created by directing the radiation from a point between the ramus and the spine on the side opposite the area to be examined to a point just anterior to the area of interest. The vertical angulation is slightly negative and strikes the film at an oblique angle. The horizontal angulations should be perpendicular to the horizontal plane of the film.

❏ **Exposure variables.** Lateral oblique projections are usually exposed with a target-film distance of 14 in at 65 kVp and 10 mA. Follow the manufacturer's guidelines for the type of film used for exposure times.

J. Lateral Skull Projections

Lateral skull projections are used to assess the entire skull. Right and left sides are superimposed on each other, with the side closer to the tube magnified more than that closer to the film. They are used to detect and locate trauma, disease, and anomalies in the bones of the skull.

Soft-tissue profiles may be obtained by using the lateral skull technique and special films or by using various filters to reduce the radiation by at least 50 percent.

Lateral cephalometric projections (Fig. 11-23) are used by prosthodon-

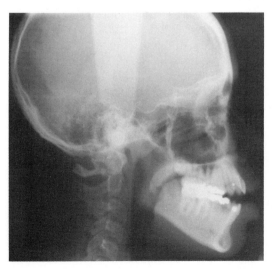

Figure 11-23. Lateral cephalometric projections are used by prosthodontists and orthodontists to demonstrate soft tissue and assess and measure growth patterns (From Miles DA, et al: *Radiographic Imaging for Dental Auxiliaries,* 2d ed. Philadelphia, W.B. Saunders Company, 1993. P. 183.)

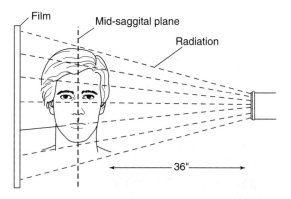

Figure 11-24. Lateral cephalometric positioning.

tists and orthodontists to demonstrate soft tissue and assess and measure growth patterns. These projections require very specific head positioning so that films taken before and after treatment provide an accurate comparison. A head-positioning device ensures accurate and repeatable head positioning. Cephalometric x-ray units are used where these projections are frequently exposed.

❑ **Film size** An 8 × 10 in extraoral film and cassette with intensifying screens is used.

❑ **Cassette position.** The cassette is positioned parallel to the midsaggital plane of the skull and centered over the zygomatic arch. At least 1 in should protrude beyond the tip of the nose (Fig. 11-24). The cassette may be held in place by the patient or a film holder. A film holder is required for cephalometric projections.

❑ **Patient position.** Position the midsaggital plane perpendicular to the floor and the Frankfort plane parallel to the floor (see Fig. 11-24).

❑ **Radiation beam direction.** The radiation is directed perpendicular to the film at the external auditory meatus (see Fig. 11-24).

❑ **Exposure variables.** The target film distance may vary from 36 to 72 in. The films are exposed at 10 mA and 65 kVp, following the film manufacturer's guidelines for exposure times.

K. Posteroanterior Projections

Posteroanterior projections demonstrate the entire skull in a posteroanterior plane (Fig. 11-25). They are sometimes exposed to supplement cephalometric projections in assessing growth and development.

❑ **Film size.** An 8 × 10 in extraoral film and cassette with intensifying screens is used.

❑ **Cassette position.** The cassette is placed in front of the patient's face in a cassette holder (Fig. 11-26).

❑ **Patient position.** The patient faces the cassette with the Frankfort

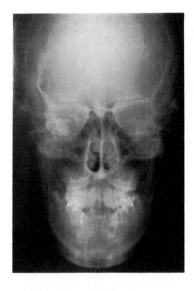

Figure 11-25. Posteroanterior projections demonstrate the entire skull in a posteroanterior plane. (From Miles DA, et al: *Radiographic Imaging for Dental Auxiliaries,* 2d ed. Philadelphia, W.B. Saunders Company, 1993. P. 184.)

plane parallel to the floor and the midsaggital plane perpendicular to the floor (see Fig. 11-26).

☐ **Radiation beam direction.** The radiation is directed perpendicular to the film from the occipital protuberance (see Fig. 11-26).

☐ **Exposure variables.** The target-film distance may vary from 36 to 72 in. The films are exposed at 10 mA and 65 kVp, following the film manufacturer's guidelines for exposure times.

L. Transcranial Projections

Transcranial projections are one of the best ways to demonstrate the temporomandibular joint (TMJ) on a radiograph (Fig. 11-27). The *Lindblom technique* demonstrates the long axis of the condyle as well as the glenoid fossa and its relationship to the condyle.

☐ **Film size.** A 5 × 7 in cassette may be used for one exposure; however, exposures are often made of both the right and left sides in the open and closed positions. All four projections may be made on a single

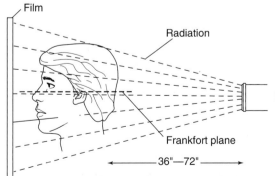

Figure 11-26. Posteroanterior positioning.

Figure 11-27. Transcranial projections. Transcranial projections are one of the best ways to demonstrate the temporomandibular joint on a radiograph (From Miles DA, et al: *Radiographic Imaging for Dental Auxiliaries,* 2d ed. Philadelphia, W.B. Saunders Company, 1993. P. 187.)

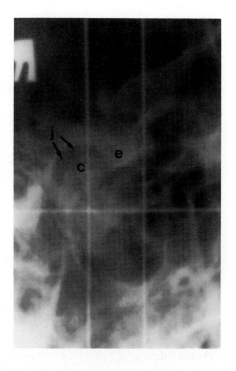

8 × 10 in cassette if lead shielding is used to protect the nonexposure areas during each exposure.

☐ **Cassette position.** The cassette is placed parallel to the midsaggital plane and against the ear and cheekbone (Fig. 11-28). Positioning devices are available to correctly position the patient, film, and radiation beam.

☐ **Patient position.** The patient is seated with the midsaggital plane parallel to the cassette (see Fig. 11-28).

☐ **Radiation beam direction.** The radiation is directed from the opposite side at a vertical angulation of +25 to +30 degrees from 2½ in above

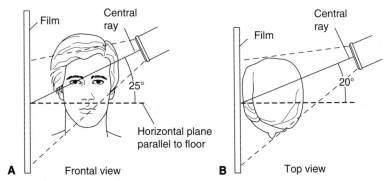

Figure 11-28. Transcranial projection positioning. **(A)** Frontal view. **(B)** Top view.

and ½ in anterior to the external auditory meatus to the condyle being radiographed (see Fig. 11-28).

❏ **Exposure variables.** The films are exposed at 10 mA and 65 kVp, following the film manufacturer's guidelines for exposure times.

REVIEW EXERCISES

1. Describe uses for occlusal radiographs.

2. Describe the technique for exposing topographic occlusal radiographs.

3. Describe the technique for exposing cross-sectional occlusal radiographs.

4. Describe the tube-shift localization technique.

5. Describe the right-angle localization technique.

6. Describe the function of intensifying screens in extraoral radiography.

7. Describe the uses for panoramic radiographs.

8. Describe the advantages and disadvantages of panoramic radiographs.

9. Describe and demonstrate the technique for exposing panoramic radiographs.

10. Describe dual, triple, and moving-center rotation panoramic x-ray machines.

11. Describe common errors seen in panoramic radiographs.

12. Describe the use and technique for the following extraoral projections:

   Lateral oblique

   Lateral skull

   Cephalometric

   Posteroanterior

   Transcranial TMJ

13. Define all the terms listed at the end of the Learning Objectives in this chapter.

LEARNING ACTIVITIES

Learning Activity 11-1: Occlusal Radiographs

Equipment:

> DXTTR trainer
> 2 size 4 films
> Round, open-ended PID

Location:

X-ray operatory and darkroom

Activity:

1. Expose a topographic occlusal view of the mandibular right posterior area.
2. Expose a cross-sectional occlusal radiograph of the mandible.
3. Process the films.

Questions:

1. Compare the two views. How does the appearance of the teeth and other anatomic structures differ in each?
2. Why?
3. Suggest possible uses for each film.

Learning Activity 11-2: Localization Techniques

Equipment:

> DXTTR trainer prepared with a coin or other small, flat, radiopaque object taped horizontally on the lingual of the mandibular right premolars and one taped vertically on the buccal of the first molar area
>
> 3 size two films
> 1 occlusal film

Activity:

1. Expose a periapical film encompassing the mandibular right premolars and first molar with the parallel technique. Note the location of the coins.

2. Expose a second periapical film of the same area with the parallel technique, altering the horizontal angulation by 20 degrees to the mesial. Note the direction of the tube head shift.

3. Expose a cross-sectional occlusal film of the mandibular right side.

4. Process the films.

Questions:

1. Describe the appearance and location of the coins on the first film.

2. How does the appearance and location of the coins change on the second film?

3. In what direction did the tube head shift? Explain the coin movement in the second film using Clark's rule.

4. Describe the appearance and location of the coins in the occlusal film. Explain.

Learning Activity 11-3: Panoramic Radiographs

Equipment:

Panoramic x-ray machine
Manufacturer's instruction manual for your panoramic machine
Panoramic film and cassette
Panoramic radiograph

Activity 1:

Read the instruction manual.

Questions:

1. How many rotational centers does the machine have?

2. What is the size and shape of the focal trough?

3. Describe proper patient positioning in the machine.

Activity 2:

1. Disinfect and prepare the panoramic machine for a patient.

2. In the darkroom, under proper safelight conditions, place the panoramic film in the cassette.

3. Correctly position and shield a student partner for a panoramic radiograph, and explain the procedure. *Do not expose the film. Operate the machine without radiation.*

Activity 3:

Name the numbered structures in the following diagram on the appropriate lines below.

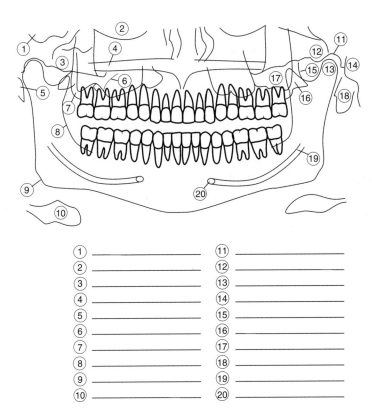

①	_____		⑪	_____
②	_____		⑫	_____
③	_____		⑬	_____
④	_____		⑭	_____
⑤	_____		⑮	_____
⑥	_____		⑯	_____
⑦	_____		⑰	_____
⑧	_____		⑱	_____
⑨	_____		⑲	_____
⑩	_____		⑳	_____

Activity 4:

Locate the following structures in the radiograph below.

Middle cranial fossa	Glenoid fossa
Orbit	Articular eminence
Zygomatic arch	Mandibular condyle
Palate	Vertebra
Styloid process	Coronoid process
Septa in the maxillary sinus	Pterygoid plates
Maxillary tuberosity	Maxillary sinus
External oblique line	Earlobe
Angle of the mandible	Mandibular canal
Hyoid bone	Mental foramen

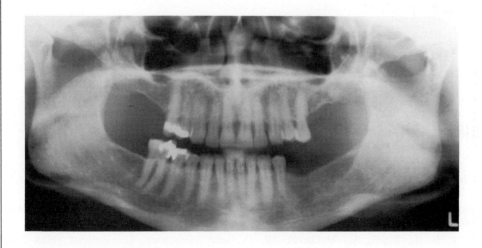

Learning Activity 11-4: Extraoral Radiographs

Equipment:

Extraoral film cassettes

Cephalometric x-ray unit

Film holders

Activity:

Correctly position the patient, film, and radiation beam on a student partner for the following projections. *Do not expose films on student partners!*

Lateral oblique

Lateral skull

Lateral cephalometric

Posteroanterior

Transcranial

Question:

Identify uses for each of the preceding radiographs.

BIBLIOGRAPHY

De Lyre, Wolf R., and Johnson, Orlen N.   *Essentials of Dental Radiography for Dental Assistants and Hygienists,* 4th ed. Norwalk, Conn., Appleton and Lange, 1985.

Frommer, Herbert H.   *Radiology for Dental Auxiliaries,* 5th ed. St. Louis, Mosby–Year Book, 1992.

Gibbs, S. J., Pujol, A., McDavid, W. D., and Welander, U.   Patient risks from rotational panoramic radiology. *Dentomaxillofac. Radiol.* 17:25–32, 1988.

Goaz, Paul W., and White, Stuart C.   *Oral Radiology: Principles and Interpretation,* 2d ed. St. Louis, C.V. Mosby, 1987.

Manson-Hing, Lincoln R.   *Fundamentals of Dental Radiography,* 3d ed. Philadelphia, Lea & Febiger, 1990.

Miles, Dale A., Van Dis, Margot L., Jensen, Catherine W., et al.   *Radiographic Imaging for Dental Auxiliaries.* Philadelphia, W.B. Saunders Company, 1989.

Radiographic Interpretation

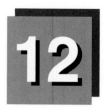

After completing this chapter the student will be able to

1. Identify the following in a dental radiograph:

   Enamel

   Dentin

   Pulp chamber

   Periodontal ligament
   space

   Lamina dura

   Amalgam

   Gold

   Stainless steel

   Gutta percha

   Silicate

   Composite

   Hypercementosis

   Supernumerary teeth

   Cervical burnout

   Calculus

   Carious lesions

   Overhanging restorations

   Apical lesions

   Impacted teeth

   Bone loss (horizontal,
   vertical)

   Triangulation

   Crestal irregularities

   Alveolar bone changes

   Root resorption

   Condensing osteitis

   Dilaceration

   Tooth and root fractures

2. Describe the best method of detection and the radiographic appearance of:

   Proximal caries

   Occlusal caries

   Buccal and lingual caries

   Root surface caries

   Recurrent caries

3. Describe the significance of and use the following criteria in evaluating periodontal disease in radiographs:

   Alveolar crest location

   Alveolar crest appearance

   Direction of bone loss

   The crown/root ratio

   The interproximal space

> Root morphology and
>   length
> Furcation involvement
> 4. Define the following terms:
> Generalized
> Localized

Marginal fit and shape

Calculus

I. NORMAL RADIOGRAPHIC APPEARANCE

Dental radiographs are used in combination with the clinical examination to identify pathologic conditions and anomalies. Careful exposure and processing technique will avoid errors that inhibit the interpretation of the radiographs. The parallel technique is preferred because it produces radiographs that most accurately represent structures.

Normal radiographic appearance of the tooth and surrounding anatomic structures must be understood before one can identify anomaly or pathology.

A. The Tooth   *outside white cap.*

❏ The *enamel* covers the crown of the tooth and appears lighter or more radiopaque than the underlying dentin because it is the most dense substance in the body (Fig. 12-1). *The enamel should appear unbroken by any radiolucencies* (dark areas) *to the cementoenamel junction* (CEJ).

❏ The *cementum* covers the root surface and is not visible radiographically because it is a thin layer with a density similar to that of the dentin that lies beneath it.   *somewhat radiopaque (very thin)*

❏ The *dentin* underlies the enamel and cementum. The junction between the enamel and dentin is distinct because of their different densities.

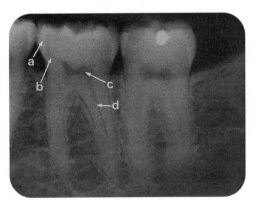

Figure 12-1. Normal radiographic appearance of the tooth. (a) Enamel. (b) Dentin. (c) Pulp chamber. (d) Root canal.

> *The dentin should appear smooth and unbroken by radiolucencies except for the pulp chamber and root canal(s).*

❏ The *pulp chamber* and *root canal* are made up of soft tissue and appear radiolucent. The size of the pulp chamber will vary from individual to individual. The root canal also will vary in appearance. The apical foramen and apical 2 to 3 mm of the canal may or may not be visible. In developing teeth, the pulp chamber and canals are quite large, the roots may be incomplete, and the apex may be surrounded by the radiolucent dental papilla. *The pulp chamber and root canal should not contain radiopacities.*

Cervical burnout may be apparent as diffuse radiolucent shading on the mesial and distal surfaces or as a diffuse radiolucent band in the cervical area between the enamel and the alveolar crest (Fig. 12-2). This is caused by decreased radiation absorption in this area and the contrast between it and the areas covered by enamel and bone that absorb more radiation.

B. Supporting Structures

❏ The *lamina dura* is the radiopaque line that follows the roots of the teeth (Fig. 12-3). Its appearance varies depending on root configuration and the angulation of the x-ray beam. It may appear well defined or nonexistent. In areas of occlusal stress it will appear thicker and more dense. *An interrupted or absent lamina dura in the absence of other signs and symptoms is not necessarily indicative of pathology.*

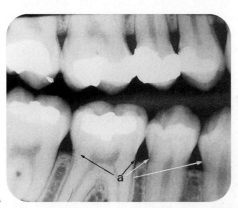 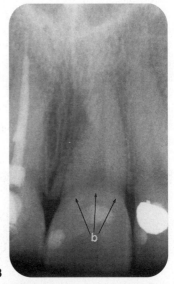

A   **B**

Figure 12-2. Cervical burnout. **(A)** Diffuse radiolucent shading on the mesial and distal surfaces. **(B)** A diffuse radiolucent band in the cervical area between the enamel and the alveolar crest.

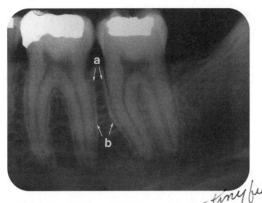

Figure 12-3. The lamina dura (a) is the radiopaque line that follows the roots of the teeth. The periodontal ligament space (b) is the radiolucent area between the lamina dura and the root surface extending from the alveolar crest around the root(s) to the opposite crest.

□ The *periodontal ligament space* is the radiolucent area between the lamina dura and the root surface and extending from the alveolar crest around the root(s) to the opposite alveolar crest (see Fig. 12-3). *The width of the periodontal ligament space varies; however, a widening adjacent to the alveolar crest or in the apical area may suggest pathology.*

□ The *cancellous* or *trabecular bone* consists of thin radiopaque plates and rods called *trabeculae* surrounding bone marrow (Fig. 12-4). It is sandwiched between the cortical plates of the maxilla and mandible. The density and pattern of the trabecular bone will vary from individual to individual; however, in general, *the trabecular pattern of the maxilla is denser and finer than that of the mandible.*

II. RADIOGRAPHIC INTERPRETATION OF DENTAL CARIES

Dental caries, one of the most common diseases seen in radiographs, begins by demineralizing the external surface of enamel or exposed cementum. It progresses by further destruction of the underlying tooth structure.

Radiographs are used to detect those carious lesions which are not easily observed in the clinical examination. Carious lesions appear as radiolucencies in the radiograph because fewer x rays are absorbed in the area of demineralization or tooth destruction. For density changes to be observed radiographically, 30 to 50 percent demineralization must have occurred. Because of this, carious lesions are usually larger than their radiographic appearance.

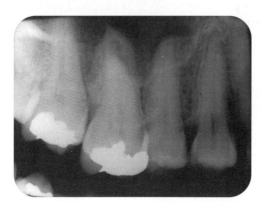

Figure 12-4. Cancellous bone consists of thin radiopaque plates and rods called *trabeculae* surrounding bone marrow sandwiched between the cortical plates of the maxilla and mandible. In general, the trabecular pattern of the maxilla is denser and finer than that of the mandible (compare with Fig. 12-3).

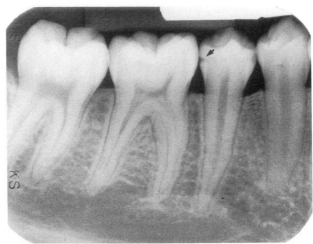

Figure 12-5. Proximal caries occur on proximal surfaces in the area from the contact point to the gingival margin. (From Miles DA, et al: *Radiographic Imaging for Dental Auxiliaries,* 2d ed. Philadelphia, W.B. Saunders Company, 1993. P. 235.)

A. Proximal Caries

Proximal caries occur on proximal surfaces in the area from the contact point to the gingival margin (Fig. 12-5).

❒ **Detection.** Proximal caries are most easily detected with bitewing radiographs or periapical radiographs exposed using the parallel technique. Anterior bitewings are less effective than posterior bitewings because of image projection geometry. The long axes of the maxillary and mandibular anterior teeth are usually angled very differently, the film is parallel to neither, and the radiation is directed perpendicular to the film but not the teeth (see Fig. 10-9). This results in the superimposition of more healthy tooth structure on the carious lesion, making interpretation more difficult. In the anterior region, periapical radiographs exposed using the parallel technique should be used to detect proximal caries.

❒ **Radiographic appearance.** The first radiographic evidence of proximal caries is a notching of the enamel, usually in the area 1 to 2 mm apical to the contact point (see Fig. 12-5). They progress along the enamel rods to the dentinoenamel junction (DEJ) following a triangular pattern. As these lesions progress into the dentin, they spread out, undermining the enamel. Their radiographic appearance becomes more diffuse as they advance into the dentin.

B. Occlusal Caries

Occlusal caries occur on the occlusal surfaces of premolars and molars, usually beginning in the pits and fissures (Fig. 12-6A).

❒ **Detection.** Occlusal caries are best detected by clinical examination. Because of the large amount of healthy tooth structure superimposed on the incipient occlusal lesion, they cannot be observed radiographically until they have progressed into the dentin.

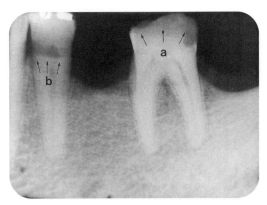

Figure 12-6. Occlusal caries (a) occur on the occlusal surfaces of premolars and molars usually beginning in the pits and fissures. They are detected best at an earlier stage by clinical examination. Buccal and lingual caries (b) occur in pits and grooves and along the gingival margin. They are best detected by clinical examination.

☐ **Radiographic appearance.** The first radiographic evidence of occlusal caries is a thin radiolucent line between the enamel and dentin. As the lesion progresses into the dentin, it becomes more diffuse. With moderately advanced occlusal caries, a thin radiopaque band of secondary dentin may be observed between the carious lesion and the pulp chamber. As the lesion becomes more advanced, the undermined enamel will collapse and all or part of the the occlusal surface and/or crown maybe missing (see Fig. 12-6*A*).

C. Buccal and Lingual Caries
Buccal and lingual caries occur in pits and grooves and along the gingival margin.

☐ **Detection.** As with occlusal caries, buccal and lingual caries are best detected by clinical examination. Because of the large amount of healthy tooth structure superimposed on incipient buccal and lingual lesions, radiographic detection is difficult before significant tooth destruction has occurred.

☐ **Radiographic appearance.** It is difficult to differentiate between buccal and lingual caries and occlusal caries radiographically (see Fig. 12-6*B*). Buccal and lingual lesions have a well-defined margin not present in occlusal lesions. The thin radiopaque band of secondary dentin which may be observed with occlusal caries will not be observed with buccal or lingual caries.

D. Root-Surface Caries *- periodontal involvement + bone loss.*
Root-surface caries occur on any surface of the root where the attachment has migrated apically and the root surface is exposed.

☐ **Detection.** Root-surface caries will usually be detected at an earlier stage with a careful clinical examination.

☐ **Radiographic appearance.** Root-surface caries follow no particular pattern (Fig. 12-7). They appear radiographically as a diffuse scooping out of the tooth structure and may be confused with cervical burnout.

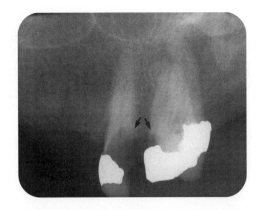

Figure 12-7. Root-surface caries occur on any surface of the root where the attachment has migrated apically and the root surface is exposed. They will usually be detected at an earlier stage with a careful clinical examination.

Root-surface caries cannot occur apical to the gingival attachment. When in question, the bone level should be assessed radiographically, and the presence of root-surface caries should be confirmed with a clinical examination.

E. Recurrent Caries

Recurrent caries occur at the margin of existing restorations.

❏ **Detection.** Recurrent lesions on the proximal and occlusal margins of restorations are more easily detected radiographically; however, large restorations may obscure early recurrent lesions. Those on the buccal and lingual surfaces are detected more easily with a clinical examination.

❏ **Radiographic appearance.** Recurrent caries appear as radiolucencies at the margin of existing restorations (Fig. 12-8). They are similar in appearance to primary carious lesions (carious lesions that occur on an unrestored surface).

III. RADIOGRAPHIC APPEARANCE OF RESTORATIVE MATERIALS

A. Silver

Silver amalgam is completely radiopaque and exhibits an irregular border (Fig. 12-9). Overhanging amalgam restorations as well as those of other

Figure 12-8. (a) Recurrent caries occur at the margin of existing restorations. (b) Existing restorations should conform to the anatomy of the tooth. Overhangs on the proximal surfaces can be identified radiographically.

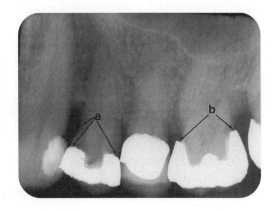

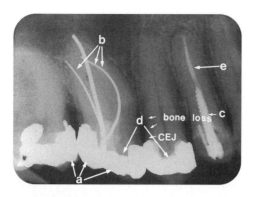

Figure 12-9. Restorative materials. (a) Amalgam. (b) Silver points. (c) Stainless steel post. (d) Calcium hydroxide base. (e) Gutta percha.

radiopaque materials may be identified radiographically on the proximal surfaces of the teeth when the restoration fails to conform to the contour of the tooth.

Silver points are also radiopaque and may be used to fill root canals (see Fig. 12-9).

B. Gold Restorations

Gold restorations are as radiopaque as silver. They may be distinguished from silver by their smooth, regular borders (Fig. 12-10).

C. Stainless Steel Pins and Crowns and Bands

Stainless steel pins and crowns and bands are radiopaque (Fig. 12-11). Stainless steel crown and bands are less radiopaque than those which are constructed of silver or gold.

D. Calcium Hydroxide Base

Calcium hydroxide base material now has radiopaque materials added so that it will appear radiopaque under restorations and not be confused with recurrent caries (see Fig. 12-9). If these materials are not added, it will appear as a thin radiolucent line and may be confused with recurrent caries.

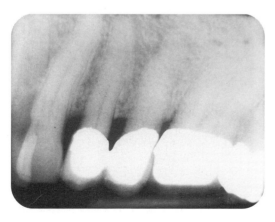

Figure 12-10. Gold crowns.

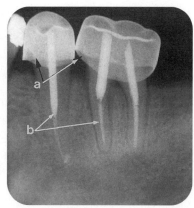

Figure 12-11. Restorative materials. (a) Stainless steel crowns. (b) Gutta percha.

E. Gutta Percha *more often seen now).*

Gutta percha is a claylike material used to fill root canals (see Fig. 12-11). It is radiopaque, but less so than metal restorative materials.

F. Silicate *~older white without fillers*

Silicate is seldom used today but has been used primarily as an anterior restorative material. It is radiolucent and can be distinguished from dental caries by its smooth, well-defined borders (Fig. 12-12).

G. Composite

Composite restorative materials are used primarily for anterior teeth (see Fig. 12-12). They are radiolucent but less radiolucent than silicate restorations. As with silicate restorations, they can be distinguished from dental caries by their smooth, well-defined borders.

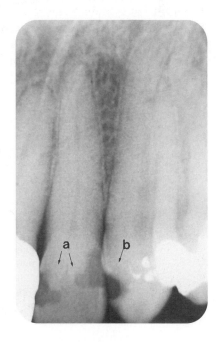

Figure 12-12. (a) Composite restorations. (b) Silicate restoration.

IV. RADIOGRAPHIC INTERPRETATION OF PERIODONTAL DISEASE

Horizontal or vertical bitewings and periapical radiographs exposed using the parallel technique are used in conjunction with the clinical examination to identify the presence of periodontal disease, assess the progression of the disease, and evaluate periodontal treatment. Radiographs also will assist in identifying factors that cause or exacerbate the periodontal condition (overhanging restorations, calculus).

A thorough clinical examination is required in addition to the radiographic examination for a complete and accurate diagnosis. Radiographs are two-dimensional images of three-dimensional objects, making it difficult to evaluate buccal and lingual bone levels because of the superimposition of the tooth and bone. In addition, significant bone loss must occur before it is visible radiographically. Radiographs cannot identify the soft-tissue changes that occur in the presence of periodontal disease. Current radiographs should be used during the examination for reference and correlation with clinical findings. Prior radiographs are useful in evaluating disease progression.

The following observations should be made when interpreting radiographs for periodontal disease.

A. The Alveolar Crest

The *alveolar crest* should be parallel to a line drawn from the CEJ of one tooth to that of the adjacent tooth and approximately 1.5 mm from the CEJ (Fig. 12-13). The lamina dura should be continuous with the crestal bone. The following observations should be made:

❑ **Alveolar crest location.** Measure the distance from the CEJ to the crest using a periodontal probe. Note areas above 1.5 mm.

❑ **Alveolar crest appearance.** Is the lamina dura present, or does the crestal bone appear porous, indistinct, or fuzzy? *Triangulation* may be seen in the early stages of periodontal disease. It is a widening of the

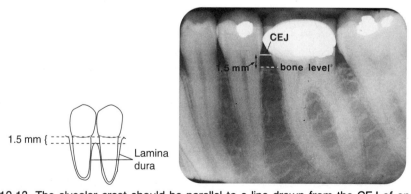

Figure 12-13. The alveolar crest should be parallel to a line drawn from the CEJ of one tooth to that of the adjacent tooth and approximately 1.5 mm from the CEJ. The lamina dura should be continuous with the crestal bone.

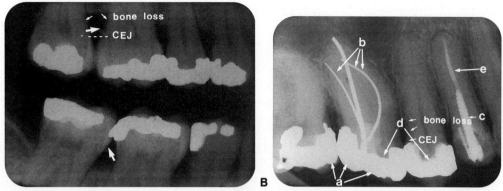

Figure 12-14. Horizontal and vertical bone loss. **(A)** Horizontal bone loss is parallel to a line drawn from the CEJ of one tooth to that of the adjacent tooth. **(B)** Vertical bone loss is not.

periodontal ligament space at the crest which is observed radiographically as a triangular-shaped radiolucency. Cup-shaped defects in the crest may be seen as periodontal disease progresses.

❏ **Direction of bone loss.** Is the bone loss horizontal or vertical?

- *Horizontal bone loss* is parallel to a line drawn from the CEJ of one tooth to that of the adjacent tooth (Fig. 12-14). It may be **localized** (confined to a specific area) or **generalized** (occurring throughout the mouth). It is the result of even bone loss.

- *Vertical bone loss* is not parallel to a line drawn from the CEJ of one tooth to that of the adjacent tooth. It may be localized or generalized but is most often localized. It is the result of uneven bone loss.

B. The Crown/Root Ratio

The crown/root ratio is one measure of the amount of bone that supports the tooth (Fig. 12-15). It is the ratio of the amount of root in bone to the amount of tooth (root and crown) not covered by bone. The prognosis is better when more root is supported by bone than tooth structure not covered by bone. A probe may be used to make measurements determining crown root ratio.

For example,

1. If 6 mm of root is surrounded by bone and 12 mm of tooth is not, the crown/root ratio is 6:12 or 1:2.
2. If 8 mm of root is surrounded by bone and 8 mm is not, the crown/root ratio is 8:8 or 1:1.
3. If 12 mm of root is surrounded by bone and 6 mm is not, the crown/root ratio is 12:6 or 2:1.

The prognosis for tooth 3 is better than for tooth 2, which is better than for tooth 1.

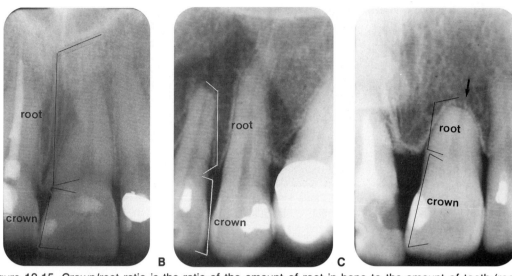

Figure 12-15. Crown/root ratio is the ratio of the amount of root in bone to the amount of tooth (root and crown) not covered by bone. The prognosis is better when more root is supported by bone than tooth structure not covered by bone. For these teeth, the prognosis gets increasingly worse as you move from **(A)** to **(B)** to **(C)**.

C. The Interproximal Space

The interproximal bone provides support for each adjacent tooth (Fig. 12-16). A wide space filled with supporting bone provides more support than a narrow one. Assess the density of the supporting bone. Bone porosity, absence of the lamina dura, and a roughened surface may be signs of bone loss.

D. Root Morphology and Length

The root is the tooth's anchor in the bone (Fig. 12-17). Long, broad roots provide better anchors than those which are short or thin. Molar roots which are close together or fused provide a weaker anchor than those which are widely spaced.

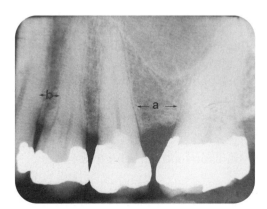

Figure 12-16. The interproximal space provides support for each adjacent tooth. A wide space (a) filled with supporting bone provides more support than a narrow one (b).

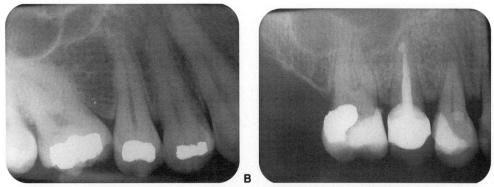

A   B

Figure 12-17. Root morphology and length. The root is the tooth's anchor in the bone. Long, broad roots **(A)** provide better anchors than those that are short or thin **(B)**.

E. Furcation Involvement

Furcation involvement must be confirmed clinically (Fig. 12-18). It should be suspected when radiolucencies are apparent in the furcation area of mandibular molars. Furcation involvement in maxillary molars is more difficult to interpret because the palatal root obscures the furcation area. If bone loss is apparent interproximally apical to the level of the furcation or if furcation arrows (triangular radiolucencies on the mesial or distal surfaces of maxillary molars which point to the furcation area) are present, furcation involvement should be assessed clinically.

F. Marginal Fit and Shape

Existing restorations should conform to the anatomy of the tooth. Overhanging restorations trap bacteria and plaque and create or exacerbate periodontal problems. Overhangs on the proximal surfaces can be identified radiographically.

G. Calculus Deposits

Calculus deposits can be observed radiographically only when they are moderate to heavy. They appear as radiopaque spurs or lumps on the proximal surfaces of the teeth (Fig. 12-19). Buccal and lingual calculus may appear as an irregular radiopaque line.

Figure 12-18. Furcation involvement should be suspected when radiolucencies are apparent in the furcation area of mandibular molars. Furcation involvement should be assessed clinically in maxillary molars if bone loss is apparent interproximally apical to the level of the furcation or if furcation arrows are present.

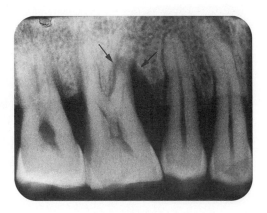

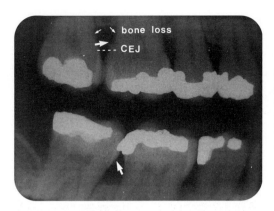

Figure 12-19. Calculus deposits appear as radiopaque spurs or lumps on the proximal surfaces of the teeth or as an irregular radiopaque line on buccal and lingual surfaces.

IV. RADIOGRAPHIC INTERPRETATION OF OTHER COMMON PATHOLOGY AND ANOMALIES

A. Apical Lesions

Apical lesions appear radiographically as spherical radiolucencies (Fig. 12-20). The border may be well-defined and radiopaque or nonexistent and porous in appearance.

B. Hypercementosis

Hypercementosis is the formation of excess cementum on the root surface which thickens the root in the area of buildup (Fig. 12-21).

C. Tooth and Root Fractures

Tooth and root fractures appear as irregular radiolucent lines on the crown or root (Fig. 12-22).

D. Dilaceration

Dilaceration is a distortion in the shape of the root or crown (Fig. 12-23).

E. Root Resorption

Root resorption may be the result of trauma or pathology. It may occur internally or externally (Fig. 12-24).

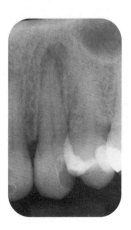

Figure 12-20. Apical lesions.

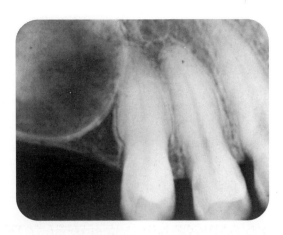

Figure 12-21. Hypercementosis. (From Haring JI, Lind LJ: *Radiographic Interpretation for the Dental Hygienist*. Philadelphia, W.B. Saunders Company, 1993. P. 154.)

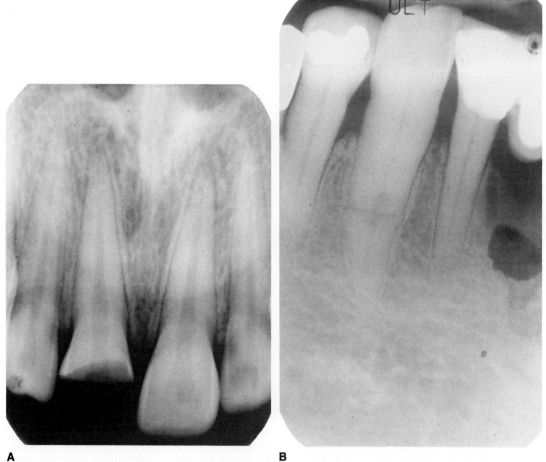

A   **B**

Figure 12-22. **(A)** Tooth fracture. **(B)** Root fracture. (From Haring JI, Lind LJ: *Radiographic Interpretation for the Dental Hygienist*. Philadelphia, W.B. Saunders Company, 1993. P. 141.)

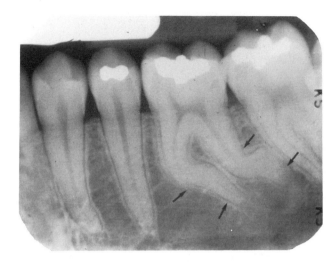

Figure 12-23. Dilaceration. (From Miles DA, et al: *Radiographic Imaging for Dental Auxiliaries,* 2d ed. Philadelphia, W.B. Saunders Company, 1993. P. 250.)

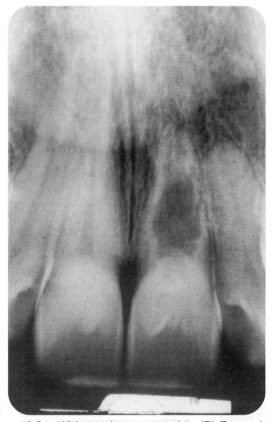

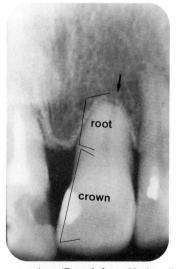

Figure 12-24. **(A)** Internal root resorption. **(B)** External root resorption. (Part **A** from Haring JI, Lind LJ: *Radiographic Interpretation for the Dental Hygienist.* Philadelphia, W.B. Saunders Company, 1993. P. 146.)

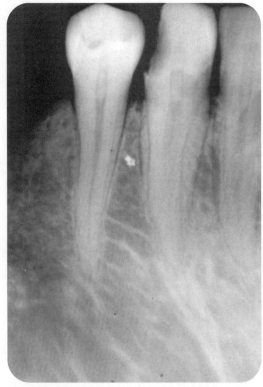

Figure 12-25. Pulp stones/calcifications. (From Haring JI, Lind LJ: *Radiographic Interpretation for the Dental Hygienist.* Philadelphia, W.B. Saunders Company, 1993. P. 149.)

tooth turns pink

❏ *Internal root resorption* appears as a widening of the root canal which can ultimately reach the outside surface of the tooth. Its cause is unknown.

❏ *External root resorption* may be the result of trauma, orthodontic treatment, or pathology. The root resorbs from the apical area, which may have a smooth or rough appearance.

F. Pulp Stone or Calcifications

Pulp stone or calcifications appear as radiopacities in the pulp chamber or root canal (Fig. 12-25).

G. Condensing Osteitis

Condensing osteitis occurs when the alveolar bone condenses in response to trauma or pathology. The bone appears more radiopaque, and there is a decrease in the size of the trabecular spaces (Fig. 12-26).

H. Impacted Teeth

Impacted teeth are unerupted and often malpositioned (Fig. 12-27). Third molars are the most common impacted teeth. Localization techniques (see Chap. 11) may be required prior to their extraction.

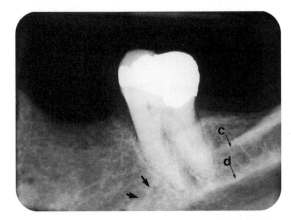

Figure 12-26. Condensing osteitis.

Figure 12-27. Impactions.

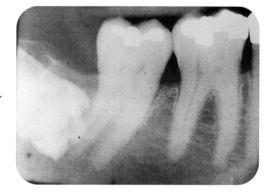

I. Supernumerary Teeth

Supernumerary teeth are extra teeth which are usually unerrupted (Fig. 12-28). The most common supernumerary teeth are mandibular premolars, maxillary incisors, fourth molars, and the mesiodens which occur between the maxillary incisors.

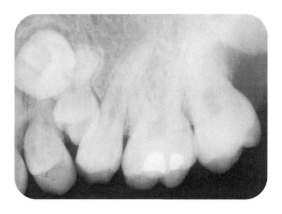

Figure 12-28. Supernumerary teeth. (From Haring JI, Lind LJ: *Radiographic Interpretation for the Dental Hygienist.* Philadelphia, W.B. Saunders Company, 1993. P. 5.)

1. Describe the best method of detection and the radiographic appearance of

>   Proximal caries

>   Occlusal caries

>   Buccal and lingual caries

>   Root surface caries

>   Recurrent caries

2. Describe the significance of and use the following criteria in evaluating periodontal disease in radiographs:

>   Alveolar crest location

>   Alveolar crest appearance

>   Direction of bone loss

>   The crown/root ratio

>   The interproximal space

>   Root morphology and length

>   Furcation involvement

>   Marginal fit and shape

>   Calculus

3. Define all the terms listed at the end of the Learning Objectives in this chapter.

LEARNING ACTIVITIES

Learning Activity 12-1: Interpretation

Equipment:

1 full-mouth survey exhibiting caries, restorations
1 full-mouth survey exhibiting advanced periodontal disease
Chart form
Charting pencils
Periodontal probe
View box

Activity:

1. Identify the following in the provided full-mouth surveys:
   Enamel
   Dentin
   Pulp chamber
   Periodontal ligament space
   Lamina dura
   Cervical burnout

2. Identify restorative materials found in the provided full-mouth surveys.

3. Identify carious lesions, overhanging restorations, apical lesions, and other noted pathology or anomalies in the full-mouth survey and chart on the provided chart form.

4. Using the full-mouth survey that exhibits advanced periodontal disease, chart bone level, calculus, and overhanging restorations, and evaluate the following (where conditions are localized, note areas):
   Alveolar crest location (measure the distance from the CEJ to the crest using a periodontal probe; note areas above 1.5 mm)
   Alveolar crest appearance
   Direction of bone loss
   The crown/root ratio (note areas where the ratio is less than 1 : 1)
   The interproximal space
   Root morphology and length
   Furcation involvement

BIBLIOGRAPHY

De Lyre, Wolf R., and Johnson, Orlen N. *Essentials of Dental Radiography for Dental Assistants and Hygienists,* 4th ed. Norwalk, Conn., Appleton and Lange, 1985.

Frommer, Herbert H. *Radiology for Dental Auxiliaries,* 5th ed. St. Louis, Mosby–Year Book, 1992.

Goaz, Paul W., and White, Stuart C. *Oral Radiology: Principles and Interpretation,* 2d ed. St. Louis, C.V. Mosby, 1987.

Miles, Dale A., Van Dis, Margot L., Jensen, Catherine W., et al. *Radiographic Imaging for Dental Auxiliaries.* Philadelphia, W.B. Saunders Company, 1989.

Index

Note: Page numbers in *italics* refer to illustrations; page numbers followed by t refer to tables.